# Praise for *Still Standing*

"Bucky Sinister is a desperately-needed tonic in this quasi-enlightened age. Sardonic, heartfelt and helpful, Bucky's writing is a lifeline for the non-spiritual."

—Patton Oswalt, comedian and author of *Zombie Spaceship Wasteland*

"Bucky Sinister has done it again: a handbook for recovery without all the gobbledygook. A personal repair manual for your psychic glovebox."

—Dana Gould, comedian

"An indispensable guide for sober misfits and those who love them. Like the best self-help authors, Bucky is insightful about everyday things we should know but don't. Probably because we were too drunk. Great stories about how to stay out of the gutter and feel okay about owning more than one towel."

—Beth Lisick, author of *Helping Me Help Myself*

"Great insight into not simply getting clean and sober, but 'living' clean and sober. Well written, easy to read, gritty and brutally honest, *Still Standing* is the book to read for anyone who desires long term sobriety or those who care for someone in recovery. Bucky Sinister hit a homerun with this one."

—Barb Rogers, author of *If I Die Before I Wake: A Memoir of Drinking and Recovery* and *12 Steps That Can Save Your Life: Real-Life Stories from People Who Are Walking the Walk*

"[Bucky's]words on the sober game are some of the most honest, insightful and illuminating. If Soberland was a nation, Bucky's books would be in the bedside drawers in every motel in the country."

—Alan Black, Scottish playwright and author of *Kick the Balls: A Bruising Season in the Life of a Suburban Soccer Coach* and co-author of *The Glorious World Cup*

# Praise for *Get Up: A 12-Step Guide to Recovery for Misfits, Freaks & Weirdos*

"[Sinister's] iconoclastic approach to addiction recovery will make a valuable addition to the growing works in this field. Highly recommended for university libraries supporting the helping professions and larger public libraries."
—*Library Journal Starred Review*

"… a brilliant piece of literary performance with poetic and savagely funny insights. The book is a wild mixture of autobiography, philosophy, social criticism, pop culture and nuttiness: the consummate self-help book for those too cool for self-help books."
—*Publishers Weekly*

"Our generation, Generation X, is a generation that doesn't like to be marketed to. We don't like to join groups and we're very suspicious of trends. In a lot of ways *Get Up* is a 12-step book for people that remember Kurt Cobain on the cover of Rolling Stone wearing a t-shirt that says, 'Corporate Magazines Still Suck.' People who think Dolittle is the best album ever made…The book's very funny."
—Stephen Elliott, *Huffington Post*

"Every single person should own Bucky Sinister's 12 step book. Addict or not. It is an incredibly funny and interesting guide on how to successfully unpack one's mind when it's overpacked. Simply put, this book should replace every magazine in every plastic surgeon's office and every bible in every motel."
—Amber Tamblyn, Emmy- and Golden Globe-nominated actress and poet

# STILL
# STANDING

# ADDICTS TALK ABOUT LIVING SOBER

# STILL STANDING

## BUCKY SINISTER

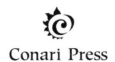

Conari Press

First published in 2011 by Conari Press,
An imprint of Red Wheel/Weiser, LLC
With offices at:
500 Third Street, Suite 230
San Francisco, CA 94107
*www.redwheelweiser.com*

4863   5410  6|12
ISBN: 978-1-57324-476-3
Library of Congress Cataloging-in-Publication Data available
upon request

Cover design by Chuck Sperry
Text design by Jonathan Friedman
Typeset in Adobe using Bauhaus 93, Myriad Pro, Adobe Garamond Pro,
and Kozuka Gothic H

Printed in the United States of America
TS
10 9 8 7 6 5 4 3 2 1

The paper used in this publication meets the minimum requirements of
the American National Standard for Information Sciences—Permanence
of Paper for Printed Library Materials Z39.48-1992 (R1997).

# DEDICATION

**People around town kept** telling me Razor was looking for me, that he was out of San Quentin. That's not the sort of thing most people want to hear. Razor was a close friend though, a friend both in our poetry lives and our drug lives. We used to get high and the next thing you know, it was three days later. We had little drug adventures that I vaguely remembered in montage sequences. We were also comrades in this strange clique of poets that my life centered around.

We were the kind of poets who shot dope in the bathrooms before going onstage, the kind that smoked crack in the alley and lost our poems, the kind that didn't get drunk so much as stayed drunk. The academics hated us and no one else liked us. We went to poetry readings where there was heckling and fights, and brought the chaos with us to other readings.

Hearing about Razor made me nervous. There was no way I could hang out with him casually with the levels of drugs and alcohol he consumed. But finally, a mutual friend told me he was clean and sober and looking for meetings. We finally hooked up and went to a meeting together.

Since then, when we talk, it's usually about our ideas on addiction, recovery, and sobriety, how two idiots like us can manage to live like clean and sober people, when we have little to no practice. We used to spend hour after hour while high and drunk, telling stories and laughing. Now, we still spend hours yakking away, only we don't need the drugs or alcohol.

It turns out we were real friends all along. It wasn't the drugs or the scene, it was true friendship. I don't have many people from that earlier part of my life anymore. It's good to have someone to count on, a solid man who's always there when I need him.

Razor, you're my brother, I love you, I'm glad I got to keep you. This book's for you.

# CONTENTS

# ACKNOWLEDGMENTS

**The last years since** *Get Up* have been full of emotions and trials. There were some people who loved that book and some who hated it. Thanks to the wonder of email, everyone tells me exactly what he or she thinks. Some offered suggestions that were anatomically impossible, even for a yoga instructor. But most asked questions and offered ideas that inspired this book. So thanks to you, the reader for constructive feedback.

There were a lot of people who aren't addicts or alcoholics but who loved the book and helped me push it on their own time and trouble: Patton Oswalt, Dana Gould, Adam Spiegelman, Jesse Thorn, and Stephen Elliott. Thanks so much, guys!

Thanks to all those I interviewed for this book, whether you ended up being included or not. Literally, I couldn't have done it without you.

Thanks to the Lucky Penny crew for all the ideas you don't know you gave me, and for helping me learn the value of fellowship in sobriety.

Thanks to my sponsor, L. for being the soccer coach when I need it and the drill sergeant when that is called for. I really will call you more often. I swear.

## INTRODUCTION

# FROM GET UP
# TO STILL STANDING

**The last book I** wrote, *Get Up,* was meant to inspire people to give 12-Step recovery another chance, or a first chance, as well as to encourage them to stick with it when it became difficult. With this book, I want to help people beyond that phase and into the next phase. Now that you've found a 12-Step group and gotten your act together, what do you do?

*Get Up* talks about the 12 steps and the misconceptions people have about how the whole thing works. *Still Standing* is for people who are already in a program of some kind and might need a nudge.

The obvious first problem addicts and alcoholics have with 12-Step programs is that they don't join. Showing up for the first time is necessary. That's the problem I tackled in *Get Up*.

The second problem that addicts and alcoholics face is that they don't stick with the program. One of two things happens here:

they relapse and are out drinking and using, or they quit going to meetings, what we call white-knuckling it.

Relapse comes in many forms. I'm fascinated with it. I've seen both newcomers and old timers go out. What makes someone relapse when they have a lot of time in a program? Why isn't the success rate 100%? Seems like somebody would have figured this out by now. If you look at how much the world and technology has changed since the advent of the 12-Step process, it's astounding. Yet we've still not come up with anything better for long-term treatment of addiction.

The relapses that are easy to understand are the ones that come when people are just a few days clean and sober, before a full detox. The physical pull is so strong. All you have to do to make it go away is get your fix, have your drink, whatever it is.

Then there are the social problems people have that make them relapse. If drugs and alcohol are in your house, it's going to be hard to stay away. If your relationships revolve around using, you're going to have trouble. If your lifestyle or your job puts you in front of drugs and alcohol, whether you're a rock star or a drug dealer, it's going to be hard on you.

The relapses that baffle me and scare me the most are the ones people have after a long time in a program. They work the steps, they attend meetings, they change their life, yet one day, they go out.

I can't find a surefire formula to explain why a person with a long time goes out. It's definitely a case by case basis. Sometimes the person can point to an event, and sometimes it just seems to happen without a reason.

After *Get Up* came out, I received a lot of emails from people who were going back after being away. Some of them were relapsed, and some were disheartened with the program of their choice. I got a lot of questions and was asked for advice on topics I didn't know about. So I, in turn, asked other people.

That's how this book came about. *Still Standing* covers the rough part of sobriety/recovery: living it. Anyone can get it in a good facility. Living it will take a strong spiritual and emotional core.

## CHAPTER 1

# GETTING SOBER VERSUS LIVING SOBER

**Anyone can get sober.** If you have the money or the right insurance, you can go to some really nice detox and rehab facilities. They'll get you sober. They'll clean you out. You'll probably even enjoy it. One of the only consistent complaints I hear from people in such programs is about having to get up early every day. People of all types have this problem: the early rising. Getting sober is not the hard part. Living sober is what's difficult. Getting through each day, getting through the rough moments, the hard patches, the trying times, that's what's hard. We hear and say in the meetings to "practice these principles in all our affairs," but what does that mean really?

Living sober is against instinct. We've learned to live drunk, high, and wasted. The way you act in a crack house is not the way you act at the DMV. The way you react to a rude asshole in a bar is not the way you react to a rude asshole at work. What we've learned in order to protect ourselves, our possessions, and our stash is not helpful to the rest of our lives; actually, acting in these ways will ruin our lives. I don't think it's the big things in life that are going to take me out. It's the little things that make me feel like I'm losing my mind. I've been through deaths and breakups and job losses sober. Love, death, and money trouble are the big three dramas in our lives. Those things are so obvious to drink over that I never would. It's such an ordinary excuse.

## Steps and Anti-Steps

When the big ones happen, that's when I get super into the program stuff. I call people. I have special themed meetings with my sponsor. I go to new meetings. I go to meetings more often. I work the Tenth Step rigorously. I divide all parts of life into two camps based on the Serenity Prayer. When the big things happen, that's when I'm at my best program-wise, which is why I don't think I'll ever relapse over one of those.

> Love, death, and money trouble are the big three dramas in our lives. Those things are so obvious to drink over that I never would. It's such an ordinary excuse.

It's like having a really sharp knife. You never cut yourself with it, because every time you pick it up, you're super careful with it. You respect the danger of the situation. However, with a dull knife, you cut tomatoes while holding them in your hand, you peel apples while watching television. That's when you cut off a finger.

The tiny traumas are what we should look out for. It's the things that get in the way of my life. Things like missing the bus, a coworker sending me a snotty email, or a friend flaking out on me can put me in a bad mindset. A car splashes gutter water on me. My shoelace comes untied in the subway station bathroom and drags through the floor, soaking up the pee of strangers from around the world. The smelly guy sits next to me on the train, then cracks open a can of malt liquor. Nothing huge in the big picture, but in the moment, those are some fucked up situations.

> **We have to do more than stop drinking; we have to learn how to live sober.**

I can easily slip into the mindset that the world is out to get me. Bad things happen to me and no one else. I can feel the world plotting against me. People are trying to get over on me. This mindset can affect how I treat every situation and person I see thereafter. This mindset usually reasons and thinks like I did when I was on a self-righteously indignant bender. It's the drunk me that a lot of people refer to as stinkin' thinkin'. Getting stuck in this headspace is what eventually takes a lot of people out. This is the hard one to shake.

This, in and of itself, is not sober behavior. Acting like a drunk is a good way to start being one again. Take the alcohol out of a drunk asshole and all you have left is an asshole. We have to do more than stop drinking; we have to learn how to live sober. The steps help us with this.

But sometimes we take steps backwards: anti-steps. We return to our defects of character, we gain resentments, we exert our will in the wrong situations, we embrace our insanity, we become un-manageable, and then we go out.

We have to do more than just put down drugs and alcohol. We have to put down the whole lifestyle. It's an interwoven life, and it doesn't work right without each piece in place.

## What Now?

There's a *What Now?* phase with recovery and sobriety. At first, what to do is really simple: go to meetings, work with others, do the steps. But something happens once life balances out, and the waters become calm. Once you've worked the steps, you've had a number of commitments, and you've helped other people through the steps, then what? It's a weird phase in which I've seen a lot of people relapse.

> It's a routine that we were in love with . . . we're busy finding the means to get our vice, getting it, using it, coming down or recovering from it, and repeating the process.

We're creatures of habit. There was some comfort in doing the same things every day or maybe every hour. It's a routine that we were in love with. Every hour is accounted for. We're busy finding the means to get our vice, getting it, using it, coming down or recovering from it, and repeating the process.

In this mindset, the bigger questions of life are all answered. The practicing addict doesn't have to think about what the purpose of life is, about the worth of the moment, or the long term consequences of his actions. But take away the immediate answer of drink or use, and the recovering addict is faced with the existential questions faced by the rest of humanity.

What now? What should I do with my life? Have I wasted my entire life? Is it too late to start over? How am I going to live outside the biodome world of rehab, meetings, and 12-Step coffee?

## The Fuck-Its

The Fuck-Its are what you have when you feel like giving up everything, especially your sobriety, over something you're going through. "Fuck it!" is what you will say before you do something really stupid.

> Recovery is too hard. Fuck it.
> Not drinking is boring. Fuck it.
> The fourth step is unreal. Fuck it.

What I've found with the Fuck-Its, is that they seem to come, not when some horrible event happens, but rather during a series of tiny ones that add up to a real hassle. It starts with missing the bus, and then breaking a shoelace, and then getting splashed by a car too close to the curb; then a random guy flashes you some attitude, and a vending machine eats your money. That's when, over the buck-fifty I put in the machine and got nothing back, I feel like drinking whiskey and killing people with an ax.

While the big ones (deaths, breakups, and money trouble) have been really hard on me at times, they are such obvious things to go out over that I don't really consider it. I immediately take action, go to meetings, and call my sponsor and friends, so I don't really see those as much of a relapse risk.

Those little things in life though, really fuck with my sense of control. They bring up feelings of "the world is fucking with me" or "there really is a God, and He's pissed at me for not believing in Him." These thoughts are a sand trap. I'll get sucked in if I set foot in it. This is why the Fuck-Its scare me much more than life's big traumas.

## AMY DRESNER

I met Amy Dresner in the mid-'90s on the spoken word scene. I ran an open mike in town, a notoriously debaucherous gathering where many people met their drug connections. People came for the pot or the speed or the heroin and they stayed for the poetry. Every summer, freaks of all types showed up in San Francisco, and many of them ended up at my event. Amy was one of those people.

Amy came from a good family in Beverly Hills. Most people think that the life she came from guarantees a good life, but for some of us, the end result is inevitable. Addiction is no respecter of social status. Amy was no exception.

Within a few months, Amy was indulging in drugs and hanging out with the other addicts. It doesn't take us long to find our kind in the world. In less than a year, Amy was back in southern California. There were various attempts at quitting and rehab before she finally gave up quitting on her own and decided on 12-Step recovery.

Since then, Amy has put her life back together. She is married to a good man and has repaired her family relationships. She's also pursuing her dreams of being a standup comedian.

The comedy world is second only to rock music for its reputation as a narcotic playground. Lenny Bruce, George Carlin, and Richard Pryor, the three men commonly thought of as the best comedians ever, all had substance abuse problems. Bruce died directly of his usage, and Richard Pryor did serious damage to himself while high, including setting himself on fire. The stories of Sam Kinison's drug use are legendary. Mitch Hedberg died as his career climbed in proportion with his drug use. Relative to these figures, the alcoholic seems tame by comparison.

Headliners of comedy clubs usually drink for free in the club. They don't always get paid that well, and they're often in town with little else to do, but the clubs are always serving alcohol. Booze softens the travel, the jet lag, and the rough nights in little towns. It's one of the few jobs where it's not unusual to drink during work hours. So how does Amy handle the comedy gig sober? How does she keep from relapsing while surrounded by free drinks? How about dealing with the competition, rejection, and personal politics that go along with it?

"Comedy is what I wanted to do my whole life," Amy told me. From a young age, watching Richard Pryor standup shows on HBO, Amy wanted to tell stories and make people laugh. But she never tried it until she was clean and sober.

Amy explains, "I was terrified. Also, drug addiction was my full time job. The [12-Step] program taught me how to show up and not let fear run my life."

She made sure she had a solid foundation in her sobriety before getting into the clubs.

"I didn't do standup at all until I had a year sober. And I'm totally out to the industry. I tell everyone on stage first thing that this is who I am. However, most people in the comedy clubs are there not only to laugh but to get fucked up. I try not to be preachy about it.

"Alcoholics have three gears: fuck you, poor me, and where's mine," Amy says.

This applies directly to the comedy world. Behind the scenes of standup is an emotional catfight of jealousy, bitterness, and envy. There's a certain amount of entitlement and self importance that a person has to have just to get up on stage, and the ones who stick with it are often rife with such personality attributes, so much so that it works against them.

Amy continues, "I'm sensitive, like all alkies. I cry. When I have a bad set, I call other comics. There are a lot of sober comics."

Amy counts her relationship with her higher power as the foundation of her career. "Comedy is a gift that's bestowed on me. I say 'God, be funny through me and I'll get out of the way.'

"When I get the Fuck-Its, I really think about the consequences of using. I'm married; it would fuck that up. I have epilepsy; I'll have a seizure if I do speed again. I just know it's not going to work. I think back to the last times I used. It always ends with me in the psych ward or the hospital. If I still feel like I have the Fuck-Its, I wait it out. I go to a meeting. I share, and it passes.

"I think back to that first year. I don't want to go through that again. It was the hardest thing I've ever done," Amy concludes.

Most of the successful comics I've met have been really nice people, but on the way to the top, there are a lot of bad attitudes, personality problems, and character defects. There are a lot of people who feel they were passed over for some superficial reason such as looks, age, or ethnicity, and resent the others who made it instead. There's unhealthy competitiveness that leads to bitterness and jealousy. There's self-pity for not having the money, time, or physical looks that the comic perceives he needs to make it.

I'm not sure where these comics are picking up the dry drunk behavior, but they have it. Some of them may have alcoholic parents, but it does remind me of the phrase "seem to have been born this way." It's really creepy to watch these guys act like drunks without having a drink. But while there's plenty of negative behavior around, Amy focuses on the other sober comics and comics with positive attitudes.

## CHAPTER 2

# MORE HABITS THAN A CONVENT

**I was standing in line** with a fellow 12 Stepper in a supermarket. This homeless guy gets arrested for shoplifting a bottle of vodka in his pants. Being alkies, we're fixated on the detail that it was Royal Gate vodka, the cheapest swill they carried in the store. Being alkies with a few years sober, we consider ourselves armchair psychologists.

"Look at that guy," my friend said to me. "Poor guy's esteem is so low he doesn't think he deserves to steal anything better."

"Nah, I don't think so," I countered. "He's been drinking that swill for so long he has some kind of emotional loyalty to it. He actually wants that more than anything else."

"Hey, man," my friend yelled out to the guy being searched by a security guard. "Out of all the liquor in the store, why did you steal the Royal Gate?"

The guy looks at us like we're nuts. "Because it was on sale."

Okay, that's nothing more than a joke, and you're free to tell it like it happened to you. But the reality is that we were one of the two addicts: the one who does whatever's cheapest and most available, or the one who does the same stuff every time.

I loved the consistency of alcohol. It's in the same place during the same hours for the same price every day. A pint bottle is the same size every time you get one. It's never cut with something else. There's always more when you run out.

> **I loved the consistency of alcohol. It's in the same place during the same hours for the same price every day. There's always more when you run out.**

I hated when the drugs ran out, trying to get more. It is fun when it shows up in front of you, when someone you know has an eightball of coke or a bag of pills or whatever, but trying to find more when that runs out was maddening to me. It would cost different prices; it would be of varying strength; I couldn't take it. I couldn't even enjoy the good stuff because I would retroactively resent every time I'd gotten lesser quality stuff in the past.

I liked doing the same thing every day, even when it wasn't fun. It was the same, and there was something comforting about that to me. After a chaotic childhood, it was nice to feel like I had control of the world, even if that world was a fifth of whiskey and watching TV.

We love the routines of acquiring, using, and recovering. It answers so many questions in our lives. There are three things to do, and we can do them over and over.

# Ten Things Every Recovering
# Addict Should Have

We're creatures of habit. Even the word *habit* is commonly used in conjunction with drug use. Drug habits. Habitual users. But it's beyond using. It's habitual living.

We have habits that are associated with our drug and alcohol use. They're not all so easy to see as the habits that are directly related. There are life choices we make that are made because they help us live the addict's lifestyle. We may think they're not related, but they are.

As I look around my writing space right now, all I see is clutter. This is something I've tried to overcome several times in sobriety, but I've had better luck quitting smoking than becoming a tidy and organized person. Mind you, when I was out, this problem was much worse. But it's still not where it needs to be for a man of forty.

I've fixed a few things along the way, things that didn't seem like much at the time, but once I made the change, I felt like I had cheated myself for years. So hopefully the clutter problem gets whacked into shape when I take the plunge and buy some real grownup furniture.

> After a chaotic childhood, it was nice to feel like I had control of the world, even if that world was a fifth of whiskey and watching TV.

I have problems with certain habits and undoubtedly you have problems of your own. Here are habits you should get, habits you should break, and habits of normal people that will amaze and astound you.

## Socks and Underwear

There's some weird thing that happens with addicts and their undies. It's one thing to not wash your jeans or your jacket; it's another thing to not wash your socks. We get used to being in utter filth. When you're fixing with puddle water or flat Faygo, having worn the same underwear for a few days is a nonissue.

But it's still gross. Not as gross as many of the other things that accompany addiction. Not as gross as abscesses. Not as tragic as meth mouth. Not nearly as unsanitary as the trash cans of vomit around the room or crapping in a bucket in the corner of the squat.

But you're not a junkie anymore. And even though you've made progress and you're much cleaner than you were, you still have a way to go.

> **When you're fixing with puddle water or flat Faygo, having worn the same underwear for a few days is a nonissue.**

I've known junkies who had trench foot, a foot disease common with the soldiers in the trenches of World War I. It was known as jungle rot in the Viet Nam War. The medical name for this is immersion foot. It happens if you never take your boots off for weeks. Prolonged exposure of the feet to damp, cold conditions can cause it. It can lead to gangrene.

Buy some new socks and underwear and throw all the old ones out. Guys, you probably still have some tighty whiteys your mom bought you in high school. They have to go.

Change begins on the inside, and right next to your insides is your underpants.

We get so strange with our money while using that our idea of essentials gets all out of whack. I didn't have enough money for socks because that would supersede my whiskey money. Which leads me to the next thing on the list:

## More Than One Towel

You have one towel that's seen better days. You use it and hang it up somewhere, over the closet door or on a hook, and you let it dry to be used the next day. I hope you're showering every day. That towel holds its shape. When you take it off the closet door, it keeps the dent. Your philosophy is that if you're clean when you use it, it's clean all the time.

> **Change begins on the inside, and right next to your insides is your underpants.**

Towels aren't that expensive. I got four for $20 at a department store. It's a small expense that made mc feel a lot more like a normal person. Get yourself a stack of new towels. It'll serve you well, especially when you have someone staying over, and you both don't have to use the same towel.

## Curtains

At the age of 32, I had never had curtains that weren't trash bags or bed sheets. That's junkie life right there. What do you think of people when you see those things in their windows? I think trash bags are tweakers and bed sheets are junkies. While you're at it, you could probably use some bed sheets, too, for your bed.

I found that discount stores like Ross, aside from having lots of clothes for sudden job interviews and weddings, has a huge home furnishings section in the back of the store. You can find all kinds of sheets and curtains back there for cheap. Before you go, there are two things you need to do.

Measure your windows and see how long your curtains will need to be. Also, find out the size of your mattress. There are standard mattress sizes: twin, full, queen, and king, and sometimes a few others like California king. The difference is a few inches in either direction, but it makes a big difference when it comes to fitting the sheets on the bed.

## Bed

When I got sober, I was still sleeping on the same lumpy futon that I had been passing out on for years. I bought that futon used from another drunk for twenty bucks. Between that and the ratty couch that had suffered many generations of punks and cats, I slept fine with the aid of some of Kentucky's finest bourbon. But soon after getting sober, I slept at someone else's house, and that someone had a fancy mattress made from foam. I laid down on it, and eight hours later I awoke thinking I had slept for days. "What the hell?" I thought. I never slept through the night back then. I thought I had some sleep disorder that prevented me from getting a good night's rest. I did have a sleeping disorder. It was called a futon. Drinking two pints of whiskey every day made it easy for me to sleep anywhere: couches, floors, bathroom stalls, offices, at the wheel, you name it. But sober was another matter. Look, if you're spending one third of your time sleeping, make it worthwhile. Treat yourself right. Having a bed that's not right is like having shoes that don't fit. And although you may not have been able to help the shoe and bed situation before, you can now.

Buying a bed can be costly, and perhaps out of your price range when newly sober. But beds are also a pain to get rid of. Most thrift store type places won't take bedding. Your best bet is to get a secondhand one from someone in your fellowship who is getting a new one. Trust me; the used bed will be better than what you've been sleeping on. A couple who has just moved in together is likely to be getting rid of one of their beds.

> **A mattress on the floor is a vestige of drug life. Outside of a creepy drug house, it looks, well, creepy.**

A mattress on the floor does not count as a bed. That is nothing more than a mattress on the floor. It's regal in a squat, perhaps, but you can do better. A mattress on the floor is a vestige of drug life. Outside of a creepy drug house, it looks, well, creepy.

One more tip: Buying a bed is like buying a car. You don't have to pay retail. The price is negotiable. Get a good price, then comparison shop. I saved up $500, and then went from place to place asking what I could get in a full size mattress and box spring for that price, including tax and delivery. Anyone who couldn't play ball got a walkout from me. I finally found a mattress marked down from $1,000 to $750, and they gave me that one for $500.

## More Than One Set of Sheets

Once you have the new bed, get some sheets. By no means should you sleep on that bare mattress. You shouldn't be sleeping on a bare mattress unless you're living in a squat or in the back of a van, and you shouldn't be doing either one of those things.

Really, you need some bed sheets. Stop sleeping on the bare mattress. You're going to spend some money on the bed. Now spend a little more and protect your investment.

Most discount stores sell sheets. You should know what size your bed is before you go shopping. You can buy a pack that has a full set of sheets including pillowcases. If you get two sets, it's easy to keep a clean set around.

Sheets are something that no one will notice if you have them, but they will definitely notice if you don't. Aside from helping you assimilate into society, it will also prolong the life of your mattress.

Dare I mention mattress pads here? Maybe that's too much for you right now. But there's this other thing that goes between the mattress and the sheets. The human body is kinda gross and dirty. The mattress pad is your mattress' machine-washable defense against the shedding of your humanity.

## Bank Account

Get a real bank account. You're a legitimate member of society. Stay away from the check cashing and payroll advance places. You have no need for them. More on those places later.

It doesn't cost anything to set up a checking account. Shop around and find a bank that doesn't charge you monthly fees. If you can't get a fee-free account, shop for the lowest fees. These fees will be much less than what the check cashing people were taking out.

## *Credit Card*

It's hard to live a regular life in this country without a credit card. Many jobs require hotel stays, and you will be asked to leave a card for incidentals, even if you don't plan on using any incidentals. You can't rent a car or a DVD without a credit card. It's likely, however, that you won't be able to get a regular card.

Once you have a bank account, talk to a bank officer about getting a secured credit card. You must leave a deposit, which they will put in an interest-drawing savings account, and the bank will give you a line of credit. I did this with $300. I put my phone bill on an automatic payment through my credit card and then put the credit card payments on automatic payment from my checking account. This is easy enough to do. I never missed a payment.

Within six months, I was getting offers in the mail for other credit cards. Most of them weren't good deals; they came with high interest rates and big annual fees. I ignored those. But my regular payments on my secured card were reporting good news to the credit services.

After a year, the bank gave me back the deposit with interest and my secured card became a regular credit card. Every so often, they raise my limit. It's big enough now to handle all my bills.

The only warning here is that it is our tendency as addicts to max out our credit. We want to get something today and not have to pay for it. There is a consequence to this behavior. I don't rack up more debt than I can pay off at the end of the month. I don't want to pay any interest for the quick satisfaction of having a big screen TV or a nice vacation.

## A DVD Player and a TV

The point of this one is that you need to occupy your time in those weird hours. There's that weird time between a meeting and sleep that you have to fill. It's these idle hours that drove me crazy. Those are the hours that the liquor store seems really close. There are also much less dangerous, but still bad, ideas. Calling up old girlfriends who really don't want to talk to you again is one that comes to mind.

While cable TV may be out of your price range, it's not that hard to get hold of a TV and a DVD player. You probably don't realize how easy these are to come by. A lot of people have spare ones sitting around that they're not using anymore. People don't want to throw away a working TV just because they don't have a room in the house without one. When the new flat screen comes home, the old, fat, bulky TV gets retired to a room they don't use, like a boxer getting a greeting job at a casino. They'd rather give Old Clunky away. But who doesn't have one? You.

New DVD players are only about $40. That even looks weird to type. I remember when they were $800. Used TVs are really cheap at all the thrift stores. So even if you can't find one for free, buying one won't be much.

When I first got sober, I'd go to a meeting and hit the video store afterwards. They had old movies for a dollar or two and two-day rentals.

At night, my mind was not calm in the least. I spun through past circumstances, worried about the future, and generally, freaked out about the state of my existence. I was too scattered to read, I already had a day's worth of program stuff, I didn't really want to talk to anyone, but I needed to focus attention outside of myself. Enter the high school teen movie.

## *Kitchen Stuff*

At one point I owned some pans and some silverware, but I can't remember where they disappeared to. I used to have a coffee grinder and a French press. I had bowls and glasses. Then they all went away.

I've left a lot of things behind. I'm not sure where it all went, but when I did get sober, I had nothing that belonged in a kitchen.

I lived in a series of houses and used whatever was there. During holiday season, I'd pick up the package with the bottle and the two glasses. I was drinking alone, so the second glass was for when I broke the first one or for the second day of drinking, whichever came first.

The point is to live like a normal person. After years of scoring drugs and using, it's really easy to score food in the same way. The natural inclination will be to subsist off food that you can buy somewhere else. You'll get little bags of fast food as a substitute for little bags of drugs.

Maybe you'll never be much of a cook. But you definitely can't cook without pots and pans, and you need things to eat out of. So get them. Even if you're making ramen noodles or mac and cheese, making your own dinner is a further step into normal.

## *Phone*

I don't know how 12 Step worked before the cell phone. Really. What went on? This all started before answering machines were even common. Back then, when you called somebody, they answered, you got a busy signal, or it just rang until you hung up the phone.

Get a phone. As soon as you can. Get a plan that allows for lots of texting and anytime minutes. People will call you anytime. They will call at noon, they will call at two a.m. They will call you in crisis, they will call you drunk, and they will call with inane questions.

The phone is great for those Fuck-It moments. When I'm ready to quit my job over some dumb thing that happened in the office, when I feel like getting into a fight over the slightest infringement on my pride, when I feel the shroud of self-pity coming over me, I call someone. It's that easy.


## DANNYBOY

I sometimes joke that I didn't recognize Dannyboy when he came into the group because he wasn't on fire. Dannyboy was one of those guys I always used to see with a cast on one leg one week and on the other leg the next week. But I never ever saw him slow down.

Dannyboy is one of the Dog Patch Winos. I'm not really sure how to describe them; the best I can do is to say they're like a biker gang without the bikes. They have all the hell-raising and partying without the Harleys. They drink like bikers ride.

Take any social group and pick out the craziest drunk. The one guy who, no matter how wasted he gets, seems to stay upright and

get more energetic as he goes. Now take one of those guy.
all the social groups you know and make them hang out with ea.
other. That's the Dog Patch Winos.

I always knew when I walked into a bar in the Mission District
and saw the DPW patches on the backs of those jackets that sooner
or later, all hell would break loose. It didn't matter the time of day
or the day of the week. More than three of them together, and
things would get raw in no time.

I was genuinely surprised when I saw Dannyboy in a meeting.
It wasn't that I didn't know he drank too much; it was that I didn't
think he would ever stop. Looking back on it now, it's hard to picture him drinking anymore, as his sobriety is as serious as his partying was. Remembering him drinking is weird, like he was playing a
character or something.

Around the time I ran into 12-Step Dannyboy, I wasn't doing
that well in my sobriety. I had no sponsor, no sponsees, no homegroup, and I wasn't through the steps. I was coming off a nasty
breakup, and I was white knuckling as bad as I had since I came
in. I was hating being sober, but I didn't want to go back to being
a drunk; then again, I did like the idea of going to Reno and getting drunk for a week and not telling anyone. But while I wasn't
yet through all the steps, I was hanging on to the first three as if my
life depended on it.

I knew I was powerless over alcohol, and I knew that even
drinking for a week would set me off in a dangerous downward
spiral. The idea that I wasn't looking to go out and get wasted for
one night was a big warning sign to me. My idea of getting drunk
once lasts for a week. I was sober enough to see the insanity there.

I did believe that a power greater than myself could restore me to sanity. Like, maybe in another fifteen, twenty years. It was going to take some time. There's no way that it would happen any sooner, right?

Now, I thought I had done Step Three, but I hadn't. I thought I had turned my will over, but I was really holding back. Looking back on it, I can see that as long as I didn't trust the group process and the community of drunks and addicts, I was still holding on to my will. I was tooling around with the Fourth Step, but without the surrender of will, you're probably not going to get something like that done.

I had this mindset that when people started to notice me in meetings, miss me if I wasn't there, or asked me to do a commitment, I picked another meeting and didn't go back. There are so many meetings in San Francisco, it was easy for me to get away with this for years. Dannyboy was a big part of why I stopped acting this way.

Dannyboy was at the meeting that is now my homegroup. Everyone seemed to know him already and like him. I was jealous of that. As much as I disliked the mob mentality and as much as I distrusted groups, I had that lonely part of me that wanted to belong to something. It was definitely a case of wanting what he had but not being willing to go to any lengths to get it.

> **My idea of getting drunk once lasts for a week. I was sober enough to see the insanity there.**

When Dannyboy became the secretary, he called on me first for every discussion. I had to say my name. I had to talk. I had to put up my thoughts for other people to judge. I knew they were judging me because I was judging the hell out of them, and they weren't any better than me, I judged.

Soon, people knew me. They said "Hi" to me at the meeting. They asked what other meetings I went to. They wanted to know how my life was going. Even after several years of sobriety, this was still very suspicious behavior to me. But it forced me to break my old habits.

I wanted to keep going to the meeting, but I also wanted to keep my isolated life. There was the conflict. Which part did I want more? Is one worth giving up the other? In this case, it has to be.

There was a really deep part of me that did want to belong to a group. I did want to be a part of a group consciousness. Whether it was a church group, cult members, cokeheads, punks, whiskey drinkers, art majors, acid freaks, or poets, I had given them all a try. They had all been a part of my life and let me down. Was this the one that wouldn't let me down?

In the end, the isolating me is the drunk me, and the group me is the real me. I want a community. I want people united by a cause or an idea that I also believe in. I think that's why the group won.

As soon as Dannyboy left the secretary position, I was voted in. I didn't want it. I became secretary with all the will of a tipped cow. It's like they waited till I was asleep in a field and then they pushed me over into a position of service. But that's another story.

I caught up with Dannyboy in my living room. We talked about his life tattooing as he got sober.

"Right when I got sober, an older tattoo artist—I think he was sober too—were talking about tattooing, and I was talking about tips, all the crazy shit people want to give you for tips.

"He told me, 'You got a vice man, you gotta keep that shit in check cuz this job will fucking pull your ass down; if you got a vice, you got a problem with a vice, this job has a tendency that people will exploit it.'

"It's funny because I don't remember who it was; I just remember the conversation and how true it rang. Later on, looking back, it's like, holy shit that guy was right. I think it was right when I got sober. He was just giving me a little schooling; that's how it went down.

"People want to tip you in drugs, or girls want to give you a blowjob; they'll find what you like, and they will grab on to that to get cheaper work . . . 'Hey, bro, I want to do this tattoo, but I only got 200 bucks. But I got some cocaine.' . . . 'Oh, yeah? Let's do the cocaine now, and then I'll tattoo you faster, which will make up for the time . . . .'

"In the beginning, when I was home tattooing, I totally exploited it. I was like, 'I'll do that for a six pack, some weed, and a little bit of blow.' People would be like, 'I don't have that much money, but I brought you this and this.' We'd be halfway through the tattoo, start partying, and then say 'fuck it.' There were a couple of tattoos I botched because I couldn't wait to start drinking or smoking weed halfway through the tattoo. 'Hey, let's start smoking that weed now,' and then I'm like 'what the fuck am I doing? I had this worked out in my head, and now I don't even know where I'm going. What the fuck?'

"Tattooers have to be really social to drum up work. I know a guy who's shot up in the tattoo world twice as fast as me. He goes to bars every night and has one or two drinks and passes out a stack of business cards, and then it's on to the next bar. He does this night after night. It's because of the social aspect of it.

"The bar scene is where a lot of tattoos spawn out of. That's where there's a little hindrance for me. I don't hang out in bars. I spend most of my time working, working on drawings. The difference between me and them is they might shoot up a little faster, but I'm banking on good old-fashioned hard work.

"You go to conventions; you hang out in the bars afterward with the other artists. That's where you go do your networking and make your connections. Sometimes I go to the bars and there's out of control tattooers. It's like bike messengers. They work really hard, and when it comes time to play, they're out of control. I'm attracted to that lifestyle; I liked to bust my balls, but when the time came to blow off steam, I'm setting myself on fire, jumping through windows."

Dannyboy's general advice:

"Keep it simple. I really believe in the Buddhist stuff when they say, 'When shit gets hard, keep it simple.' The harder it gets, the simpler you keep it. If you're going through hard shit, simplify your life.

"Someone asked me how you deal with the Fuck-Its. I say 'fuck it' to the Fuck-Its. I figure the two things cancel each other out. It really does work. When I used to say 'Fuck it, I'm going to go do that,' I now say, 'Fuck it, I'm NOT going to do that.'"

# CHAPTER 3

# ACT LIKE NOTHING'S WRONG

*Normal.* **That word, to** me, is like a Martian, Bigfoot, or an elf. What is normal? A lot of people think they know, but who really does? In a room full of junkies, having a set of works on you is normal. In an office building full of executives, a briefcase is normal. A junkie with a briefcase or an executive shooting up is abnormal, although these things happen. So what does normal really mean to me, and what should it mean to you?

Normal is not being an addict or recovering addict. We're not normal. We've done things that normal people will never do: drinking in the morning, scoring dope in bad neighborhoods, and taking prescription meds that weren't meant for us. Even now, we go to meetings, do step work, and reach out to struggling addicts. Normal people don't do this stuff. We're not normal, and there's no way we're going to be, but the fact is we have to live in the normal world.

In one sense, you'll never be normal again. You've done and seen things that normal people will never do. The sum total of your experiences may be equal to theirs, but the specifics will be vastly different. Most people in this country have not gotten high. That's weird to think about. In the circles that we came up in, this is not the case.

What normal means depends on where you live. The most common lifestyle around you is what is normal. There are circles of normalcy around you, concentric circles, like a target. At the center is you. The next circle around you is the people you live with, roommates or family. Outside that is your immediate community, the people who live in your neighborhood who you see at the grocery store. Outside that are rings of the rest of your city, the part of the state you live in, the rest of the state, the part of the country you're in, the country as a whole, your continent, and the world. What's normal depends on what ring you're a part of. What's normal in your hometown isn't normal in another part of the world.

> **Living like you're normal is much softer than living like you're still using. It will separate you that much further from a relapse.**

Then there's another kind of normal, a normalcy of experience. Whether you are a recovering addict, a mother, or a professional athlete, you have a set of experiences that make you like or unlike other people regardless of where you are from. What soldiers experience is normal for soldiers in all armies, whereas their experiences are abnormal for everyone else.

My point is I want you to find a normal you can assimilate, some kind of normal that exists around you. Living like you're normal is much softer than living like you're still using. It will separate you that much further from a relapse.

For years, normal for me was drinking every day. I made my world of other people who drank every day. It's not hard to build a world where that kind of drinking looks to be the norm. Who was going to tell me to quit? The other drunks in the bar? There was a line of us, all rationalizing each other's usage by example.

There's a reason they make you get up early every day in rehab. It's normal to wake up every day and go to work or take your kids to school. Many of us have not had this in our lives. The minutiae of life that normal people accept, wouldn't even think to question, becomes a big problem for us. Normal people try to build healthy routines.

The lifestyle that goes along with drug and alcohol use is foreign to most people. They've never scored drugs from a stranger. They've never seen a gun pulled on someone else. They've never even seen anyone shoot up with a needle. None of that is normal.

But there are some parts of normal that you can have. Get a job. Go to work every day. Show up on time. Pay your taxes. Have your utility bills in your own name. Those things are all part of a normal life.

## Seven Habits of Highly Normal People

*The Seven Habits of Highly Effective People* was a huge bestseller, but it was aimed at people who already have their shit together on the basic levels. In this section, I'm going to aim lower, at the ground, where you live. This is some basic normal-person type stuff to do that will help you fit into society. Everything on this list I started doing in sobriety, some of it only recently. It's helped me get along in the world. These are all things I didn't know I should be doing or thought were unnecessary.

### Saving tax forms

You know that one part of your W-2 that says it's for your records? Most people keep those and know where they are. When you apply for a mortgage loan, they'll ask you for them. You're expected to have them.

### Keeping up with world events

Normal people know and care about what's going on beyond their neighborhood. I'm terrible at this one. The further it is from me geographically, the less I care about it. If it weren't for Risk-type games that I've played, I'd have no knowledge of geography.

If David Letterman's Top Ten list covers a subject beyond my knowledge, that's a problem. They're writing towards the ignorant American, and that guy knows more than I do.

### Keeping a list of past landlords

When you get an apartment in your own name, the rental agent is going to ask for references from former landlords and their contact info. I sublet for years. At one point, I hadn't dealt with a landlord personally in over ten years. That's the San Francisco way. I gave them the leaseholder info when asked for it, and told them up front who those people were.

## Budgeting

Instead of spending money until it runs out, you can plan how much money you're going to spend on some things ahead of time. If you budget correctly, you'll never need to borrow money or get a paycheck advance, because you'll be living within your means. For drug addicts who cash a GA check, then spend the money on crack until it runs out, this idea sounds extraterrestrial.

Around the first and the fifteenth in my neighborhood in San Francisco, the days the checks came out, the usual addict-populated streets were empty. The addicts were in hotel rooms using. Within a few days, they dotted the sidewalks, and by a week, it was back to the comedown circus on Mission Street.

The addict's mindset of action without consequence is antithetical to the ideas of budgeting and saving money for later . . . which brings me to my next point.

## Saving money

In the current economy, saving isn't as common as it used to be. I know a lot of people are in serious debt these days. But for addicts, the idea of saving money is a new one. The best thing we saved was old cigarette butts in the ashtray that we were extremely grateful for when we ran out of smokes and money.

The easiest way for me to start saving money was to open a savings account at my bank. When I deposited a check, I transferred anything I considered extra into the savings account right there at the ATM. By talking to my bank, I found out that they could automatically transfer funds on a monthly basis from my checking account to my savings account, and if I did this I would have no checking account fees.

A savings account isn't going to generate very much interest. They'll give you a token amount, but it will be less than what you have in a change jar at your house. It's better than nothing, though, and it will help you manage your money. Most importantly, when life's little surprises hit you in the face, you'll have the money to deal with them.

## Investments

In early recovery, investments were the farthest thing from my mind. They sounded like fairy tale talk. You might just as well have told me that I could buy a cloud castle or shares in a rainbow. Investments definitely sound like things that other people have, a part of a world you don't belong in. I hear that word and immediately think of Gordon Gecko in the movie *Wall Street*. But there are ways to invest your money even when you don't think it's very much.

> **If you have around $5,000 a year over what you need, instead of buying a bitchin' set of rims, gold fronts, or a 60-inch television, consider opening an IRA account.**

I'm really loathe to give you any kind of serious financial advice here, aside from don't overspend with your credit cards and try to save money every month. There's a whole section of books in every bookstore about how you should invest your money, and much of that information conflicts. But I'm going to tell you about one way to invest your money that you should consider.

IRA accounts I can fully endorse. What you do with the money in the account, that's up to you. Buy another book for that. If you have around $5,000 a year over what you need, instead of buying a bitchin' set of rims, gold fronts, or a 60-inch television, consider opening an IRA account. There are two kinds of IRA accounts, the regular and the Roth, but I don't want to go too far into the differences here. If you have the money, ask someone at your bank or do your own research to see which one is right for you.

Things that are investments: buying a home, savings bonds, IRA accounts, stock market purchases, savings accounts, certificates of deposit, buying or starting a business.

Things that are not investments: tattoos, Harley parts, comic books, car speakers, limited edition DVDs, jet skis, that car you plan on fixing up and selling, and anything you bought from a TV shopping network.

## Dental work

If you know the name of your favorite tattoo artist but not the name of your dentist, you're probably a drug addict. I was in this category for a long time. Like many other addicts and alcoholics, I didn't want to go to the doctor or to the dentist because they would tell me some bullshit like "you should stop drinking." Psychiatrists, too, for that matter: "You should stop drinking and using because it's making you depressed." What do they know?

Most of the years that I was out, I couldn't afford regular dental work anyway. It's expensive for people living paycheck to paycheck.

One of my requirements when I was searching for a full-time job was that it have dental benefits. The plan was to go to the dentist once the benefits kicked in. Until then, I put off the dental care.

Then that day came when my benefits were activated. Now I had to face the fear of no regular dental visits all through the '90s and most of the next decade. It had been a long time since I had regular care.

> I had to face my fear. The first thing I did was share that at group level. And as it turns out, my fears were not special or unique.

Frankly, I was scared. I knew there was something wrong in there, but I had no idea how bad it was. I had pain off and on with my molars. Some days my breath was really bad. But still I had hesitations. I was afraid of the pain and the idea of someone poking around in my mouth with a needle, but my worst fear of all was that sound of the metal instruments scraping enamel. I also had this horrible fear of the dentist dropping the tools down my throat.

I had to face my fear. The first thing I did was share that at group level. And as it turns out, my fears were not special or unique. The only people in the group who weren't freaked out about dentists were the ones who had scammed painkillers from them. There were a bunch of people in there who had been through the same thing. I got phone numbers of people to call if I thought I would chicken out. With the knowledge that I had their support and knowing I would look like a wuss if I went back there without getting the work done, I was able to face down my fear and go to my appointment.

My mouth was a scary story that dentists tell their kids about at night. I had to have deep cleanings on four separate visits. Then two more visits to fill cavities. Shortly after that, I had a root canal and then an extraction. The only good thing I heard was that I would've lost several teeth in the coming year had I not gone in when I did. When I finally went and just had a cleaning without having to get shots, I was stunned.

## Prescription Drugs

Whether or not a drug addict can safely use prescription drugs is a touchy subject, but I'm just the guy to touch it. The problem is, I don't think there's one hard and fast rule that everyone can follow. It's a case-by-case type of situation. I can't really lay out rules for other people to abide by, so I'll give some examples from my own life.

> **I don't think there's one hard and fast rule that everyone can follow. It's a case-by-case type of situation.**

I had to go to the dentist after not having gone in over ten years. No kidding around, I was scared as could be to be in the dentist's chair. I have all kinds of weird fears surrounding dental work. I'd mention them, but I don't want them to spread to you. The dentist saw how freaked out I got as the instruments neared my mouth. He offered to give me a prescription so I could take something before I showed up to relieve the anxiety. I passed. If it was only fear, and not pain, I didn't think it was appropriate.

Some recovering addicts have told me they had all their dental work done without anesthetics. I don't see how I could've made it. It still felt like someone had hit me in the mouth with a brick by the time the work was done. I felt no euphoria whatsoever from the anesthesia. It was administered by a physician for a specific purpose.

I took ibuprofen for the pain afterwards. It was enough for most of the procedures. I waited as long as I could, then took some that would kick in and help me sleep.

I took a Vicodin prescription around the time of the root canal. I was in a lot of pain, a blinding, balance-jarring, disorienting amount of pain. It felt like an ice pick had been jammed in my jaw. I took four out of the twenty pills I was prescribed, and I only took them when I had to sleep. It was several days from when I was diagnosed to when I was able to be treated. After that, I got rid of the remainder. There are some out there who would consider those four pills a relapse. I didn't consider it one. Neither did my sponsor. I called one of my close friends in recovery who has dealt with a lot of medical procedures and talked at length with him about it.

As far as the fear goes, how did I deal with that? With the help of my community. I shared off-topic at my homegroup. The issue was of importance to my sobriety, not only to my staying sober, but to my living sober. What made my fear great was keeping it a secret. Once I shared, the fear subsided. What further helped me was finding out that everyone in the room had gone through it, or knew that it was coming up in their lives too. Someone told me to imagine it as a tattoo that hurts more than others, but is the best-looking tattoo ever; this worked well for me, although it may not work for you if you haven't gotten some painful tats.

I wrote down my specific fears of what could happen during the process of receiving dental work. I read them out loud to some other people after the meeting. They howled and laughed and talked about horror movies it reminded them of. Those fears had less weight after that. They showed themselves to be irrational and fantastic.

As far as a lot of prescriptions go, the doctors usually err on prescribing too much rather than not enough. Their main issue is that they don't want you to be in pain. What this means is you don't need all you are prescribed, and just because it is prescribed for you doesn't mean you have to take all of it until it's gone.

The key for me was being open and honest with those close to me in sobriety. Not only do you have a responsibility to your sponsor and your sponsees, but there are a lot of other people around you who count on your presence. There were people I'd barely talked to who offered me help and encouragement, and as a result, we became closer.

> You don't spell danger without anger. In recovery, it's the most critical emotion when it comes to relapse prevention.

## Anger Is Energy

Anger and the addict have a strange relationship. Anger has gotten me out of and into the worst situations of my life. You don't spell danger without anger. In recovery, it's the most critical emotion when it comes to relapse prevention.

A common story of relapses I hear involves anger escalating to rage. People have a long time sober or clean, and then something happens that makes them so mad, they find themselves hitting a pipe or sucking off the bottle. I don't hear as much about happiness or depression leading into relapses, but so often anger is an issue in relapse.

Anger is human. There's nothing inherently wrong with it. When it gets troublesome is when it supersedes our sense of action and consequence. It can make our decisions for us.

A lot of us come from violent childhoods. Anger is something we learned early and used often. Anger kept us safe at times. Anger was the way we got what we needed, and it helped us avoid what would hurt us.

The strongest physical sensation for me to drink came during a moment of rage. I was working security at a club. I remember the feeling of pure rage as I chewed out a drunk guy outside. He had been a smart ass inside, attempting to bully me into letting him break the rules. I threw him out. When strongly confronted, he totally backed down. It should've been over at that point. It didn't matter. He was outside of the club. I had done my job, but for some reason it wasn't enough. I yelled at him until he had completely walked out of view.

Rational behavior disappeared. The sane me wanted him out of the club and on his way. That happened. Then rage took out rationality, and I wanted him to try something. I wanted to fight him. I became more enraged. I felt every fighting bit of me flare up and get ready to go.

I went back in. I wanted a drink. I wanted bourbon. I could feel it in my teeth, in my gums, burning in my throat. That whiskey seemed really close. I wanted a fight, a pint of whiskey, a pack of smokes, and a gram of coke. That would get me started. Then, from there, I could expect unemployment, jail, or the hospital.

Rage is the ultimate form of self-righteous indignation. In that situation, I was right. However, I acted in a really wrong way. I felt justified since he was the asshole. But then I became the second asshole. Being right wasn't enough. I had to be beyond right. *More righterer.*

More righterer is what I call it when I'm being too stupid to know how to use the word right. It's that blind, irrational sense of "I'm right and you're fucked." Yeah, you might be right, but I'm *more righterer.*

Rage is like cocaine. It's never enough. The madder I get, the better I feel. But like drugs and alcohol, the comedown is horrible. I feel shame and self-loathing. I know I've acted like every jackass I've ever resented. For something that feels so right when it's happening, it sure feels shitty when it's done.

Rage is anger without a limit, detached from its source. Where anger is human and sometimes necessary, rage is that same anger inflated and set loose. If the target is no longer in sight, then rage will attack another target, for it needs no reason and has no sense of consequence.

Rage and whiskey go hand in hand for me. It's like cocaine and alcohol for some people, like coffee and cigarettes. One makes me want the other. I'm a hell of a lot closer to drinking after a fight than before one.

I've seen a lot of men who turn this rage outward and women who turn it inward. It works the other way around too, but those are the ways I've seen it most often. Men yell at people, get into fights, break up with their girlfriends, and wreck cars. Women internalize, hate themselves, eat or starve, and cut themselves. These are stereotypes, but they do happen a lot with addicts.

## JESSE M

I normally hear Jesse before I see him. In the train station entrances, when I hear the Johnny Cash-like voice echoing off the walls, I know it's Jesse down there playing for the spare change of the commuters. Coming around the corner, I'll see him, a man who looks nothing like the country songs he's singing. Jesse is decked out head-to-toe in hardcore punk gear. It's striking, to see the Mohawk and hear the twang together.

Jesse grew up in San Francisco's Tenderloin district, an area that it's more common to end up in than to be from. The Tenderloin was once a burgeoning theater neighborhood, but at some point it degenerated into one of the bleakest neighborhoods in the country. As is often the case in San Francisco, mere blocks from the Tenderloin is the opulence of Union Square and the bright lights of the remaining theater houses. Inside the boundaries of the neighborhood are the residential hotels and a soup kitchen. It's the last stop for a lot of drug addicts. Drug users conduct business openly on the street and get high in plain sight. From the old men waiting at the bars for them to open at six in the morning to the young suburbanites coming down to score Oxycontin, the neighborhood welcomes all those who have succumbed to addiction.

Not everyone who lives in the Tenderloin is a drug addict, but they all have to see them. Some live there for the low rent, sacrificing quality of life outside the apartment for relatively cheap square footage inside. There is no way to live in the neighborhood without dealing with addiction on some level.

I met Jesse long ago at meetings when he was a teenager. Then he went out, and I didn't see him again for a long time. Years later, he showed up again, still high but coming down, full of tears, and asking for help. Since then, he's been solid in his recovery.

One thing that's stuck out to me about him is his compassion toward the down and out. Maybe it's his upbringing in the sad neighborhood in which he still lives, or maybe he just has a big heart. He's a nonjudgmental guy who will offer his help to anyone in need, as if he or she is an equal. While I've seen many shy away from the hard case newcomers who are dirty, smell bad, and look a little crazy, Jesse's always in there, offering his friendship.

I talked with him on a lazy afternoon. He called me to talk about performing and standup comedy. We soon got into a whole conversation about what people think is funny, what makes tragedy funny, and the dark sense of humor that many recovering addicts have. Then we talked about relapsing.

"I've been in and out since I was fifteen. Boredom is the number one cause of relapse. When I'm bored, I play music, hang out with friends, goof off, anything to keep my attention for five seconds. I can act out in other ways that don't involve drugs and alcohol.

"Also, when a good lookin' gal with a bottle of booze would want to drink with me, that was hard for me, too. My first girlfriend was like, 'Those people have you brainwashed. You can have one drink.' And between me wanting her and my resentment against being an alcoholic, I bought into it.

"I had a lot of resentment against being in the program, I had a big case of the boo-hoos: poor me, I'm eighteen and I'm sober, and everybody else is partying.

"Relapses, for me, are dangerous. I'm not the guy who's going to go to prison or end up homeless. I'm a manic-depressive alcoholic. If I relapse, there's a good chance I'm going to commit suicide. Suicide isn't a good option. If I want to keep sane, coffee and cigarettes are as much as I can do.

"Now, being a doorman, I'm around booze all the time at my job. I make sure to tell everyone there that I'm an alcoholic, so in case I do weaken, have a bad day, and break down and ask for something, they won't serve me.

"Being a doorman actually reinforces my recovery. I see drunks around me all the time, acting stupid. For me, seeing drunk idiots is a good reminder of what it's really like. It's easy to fantasize about drinking whiskey, but when you see a guy with the DTs, you're like, maybe not today.

"Sometimes I see the bottle of whiskey and I want it. But then I think of it like it's a bottle of bleach. I picture myself pissing out my ass and shaking and wondering why everyone hates me. That's the reality of what drinking does to me."

## Relapse versus Reality

I like this idea of the fantasy of the relapse versus the reality. Most people who relapse think they have it under control now, or they are "better." I tried everything short of stopping completely: stopping drinking hard liquor, not drinking in bars, not drinking until after a certain time, not drinking after a certain time, only drinking on special occasions. These never worked. I won't be fooled into thinking they will after being sober for any amount of time. But I think people do fool themselves with ideas like these.

Jesse also talked about boredom. Boredom is a killer. When I first got sober, I didn't know what to do after 8 p.m. That was always taken care of during my drinking and using years. If I wasn't wasted by then, I was figuring out how I would be before the end of the night.

I needed something to do. This was around the time people were making the transition from VCRs to DVD players, and someone sold me a VCR and a small TV for almost nothing. I got a membership at my local video store, which was on the walk back from the two main places I went for meetings. There were days when I didn't feel like going to meetings, but I burned that routine of a meeting and a movie in my brain. This worked for a while.

> **Boredom is a killer. When I first got sober, I didn't know what to do after 8 p.m. That was always taken care of during my drinking and using years.**

I thought about what I liked to do before I started drinking. There were the movies, and I had taken care of that. In high school and college, I had been in a few plays. One of the things I didn't like about plays in college is that they seriously cut into my party life. They took up way too much time.

It didn't take long to get into a small local production. In San Francisco, if you want to perform for free, you can do it easily. Making a living in the arts is really difficult, but participating is easy. I got a part in a play that took up four nights a week of my time. I was able to use my obsessive skills to learn my lines and really dive into the play.

Not everyone is artistically inclined. There are plenty of things to do other than the arts. I know a lot of guys who buy an old Harley-Davidson that needs constant tinkering to get it running and keep it running. Some of them buy two so that one runs while they are working on the other one. It's also common to take classes. There's any number of things to do. Get a hobby. Nerd out. Become a gearhead. Get your degree. Learn a trade.

> **There's any number of things to do. Get a hobby. Nerd out. Become a gearhead. Get your degree. Learn a trade.**

In my drinking days, I worked at a bar for seven years. I worked the door, barbacked, booked entertainment, and tended bar a few nights. I genuinely liked it, but I never got paid very well doing it. However, it gave me perks, mostly club courtesy at other bars, where I got in for free when there was a cover and got to stay after hours and drink with the staff. I realized later that, more than the drinks, I liked the camaraderie and being behind the scenes.

I don't have to give up any of these things in my life. I know that's what I should include to keep myself happy. It's not only work and my social life where it comes into play, it's also the meetings. I love hanging out with the others after a meeting at a diner or café. At my homegroup, I love being a part of the business meetings and having a commitment.

Since getting sober, I've done security work for a variety of people and clubs. I still keep one door gig a week. I do like the work, and now I get to hang out at a club without feeling like I have nothing to do there. Since becoming sober, I find most clubs boring. Working gives me something to do between stage acts. It's also a good way to carry the message to those who still suffer. I'm a gateway to meetings for the drunks and addicts who hang out where I work. There are a lot of performers who come through town who are 12 Steppers looking for a meeting. It's a lot easier to get to a meeting out of town when you have a buddy to go with.

# CHAPTER 4

# HITTING WALLS

**Marathon runners have what** they call The Wall. They also have runner's high. We know what the high is. They bottom out on exhaustion and exertion, and they get high. The Wall, for them, is when the glycogen levels are depleted and the body has to turn to fat burning for energy. Usually this happens around mile 20. I think around mile 2 is when I would hit that wall. My point is, the wall is when they are faced with a decision: quit or continue. Their body tells them they are done and it's time to give up. Using an inner resolve and a strength of will, they push on, not wanting to lose all they've worked for so far.

We have walls in recovery as well. Our walls aren't physical, but spiritual. We have walls that we must scale to get to the next development of our spiritual selves.

While working the steps, it's really obvious to us what we need to do next. As soon as we figure out one step, there's another looming in the distance. It seems insurmountable, but one way or another we find our way over the wall, to find another wall that is more ominous than the last.

As a drunk, every day was figured out. I knew what I was doing. Wake up. Get to work. Get out of work. Drink. Repeat. Weekend? Wake up. Go to store. Buy whiskey. Go home. Drink. Repeat. The walls in this are: I'm at the bar and out of money, or I'm at home and just ran out of whiskey.

> **Our race is our life. We don't get to one point where we are better, or are recovered fully; we have our addictions for our lifetime.**

Now, when I get off work, there's a choice waiting for me. Do I stay home and write? Do I go out and see a movie? Do I call up the girlfriend for a date? What I do is up to me. I'm not following a bottle around town.

In the big picture, not knowing what's next is hard for me to handle emotionally and spiritually. I get really discouraged not knowing what my next move should be, even when there's nothing wrong. Should I go to grad school, or should I get a better job? Luxury problems, really.

It's also not clear what to do next program-wise. Should I do Steps 10 through 12? Get another sponsee? Do another commitment? Go through the steps again with a new sponsor?

The whole idea runners have about The Wall is that once they get over it, they are free to run and finish the race. Here's how the metaphor applies to us: Our race is our life. We don't get to one point where we are better, or are recovered fully; we have our addictions for our lifetime.

We need to switch from seeing obstacles to overcome to feeling inspiration and excitement from our ability to live our lives free of the obsession to use.

We don't have a runner's high. We have a pink cloud. But the pink cloud is only for newcomers, right? Not necessarily. You have multiple pink clouds in your life.

### VOLTMETER

Voltmeter is a 50-year-old health care professional. He has four years sober.

"I'm in a 12-Step group for the simple reason that I had thirteen years sober but eventually relapsed with Herculean repercussions. Why relapse? Complacency. 'I have this under control,' I kept telling myself. I also didn't attend meetings, didn't have a sponsor or a network of people in recovery. In short, I had no program. Without a program, I couldn't stay clean. I tried switching drugs with even worse effect. Desperation eventually (four and a half years later) drove me to a moment of clarity: I realized that the pain of change was less than the pain of the same old same old.

> We need to switch from seeing obstacles to overcome to feeling inspiration and excitement from our ability to live our lives free of the obsession to use.

"Basically, I would say that my relapse was the result of many factors, with the prime one being complacency. But I can't exclude arrogance and the insane notion that I could use once safely.

"The only time that I might be tempted to use is when there is extreme stress with my wife or during one of my abysmal periods of depression. I get the Fuck-Its."

Voltmeter finds it challenging working in a detox facility. "The parade of the sick, the damaged, the hopeless, and clueless can be despairing. Add to this that, out of the whole agency, I am one of barely a handful of recovering addicts/alcoholics.

"I go to meetings. I have a network of recovery. I have a sponsor who I use to guide me through the steps. I get down on my knees in the morning and at night. I ask for help. I'm grateful for another day clean.

"Besides recovery lit, I still read Burroughs (albeit from a different perspective) because I finally realized that *Naked Lunch* wasn't about getting high, but about being dopesick and miserable. Most literature about drugs doesn't inspire me. Likewise, most movies are two-dimensional as few filmmakers have raging habits. It just seems so fucking artificial."

## Chasing After That First Recovery

We all know what chasing after that first high is like. It's been happening since the dawn of drug use. Cavemen addicts did it. Extraterrestrials on flying saucers are doing it. I don't always think it was that first high; with some drugs like LSD and marijuana, sometimes the best use is a couple of times in. But there's that peak experience that comes with, if not the first use, an early one, that is so awesome and flawless that it reorganizes our life.

I think nonaddicts have this experience too, but not the way addicts do. For us, it is much better. The world makes sense during and after the experience. Normal people might take some mushrooms at Burning Man and have a really good time, but then they go back to their normal lives. The addict thinks he's found the secret to earthly happiness, and soon his life revolves around the fungus. With us, a peak drug experience reorganizes our sense of priorities and ethics. A holistic philosophy about life, the universe, and everything emerges. Normal people just think they'll do it again someday.

Even at rock bottom, we picture our drug of choice at its best moment in our lives. I was miserable the last few years of my drinking, but I still remembered the first years when it always worked out great for me. I remembered it as making everything better rather than making it worse. I remember thinking people liked me more and that it was easier to make friends while I was drinking. I didn't recall drinking and having everyone resent me for wrecking the party. I thought of the women I met while drinking rather than the relationships I ruined because of the drinking. It's the romanticization of the experience that keeps us there.

> I thought of the women I met while drinking rather than the relationships I ruined because of the drinking. It's the romanticization of the experience that keeps us there.

I've seen some people who want the first recovery, that first pink cloud they get. They miss those early days with other short timers as well, when everyone leaned on each other heavily and went to meetings every day. Living in rehab or the SLE (sober living environment) seems so simple and welcoming after you get out in the real world and have an apartment where nothing is done for you and no food is cooked for you and no bills are paid for you. There are those revelations of the self, like when I saw that 90% of my problems were self-induced, brought on by drugs and alcohol either directly or indirectly, or when I found out that all of my close friends at the bar didn't know who the hell I was, that my entire social life there was imaginary. The first six months of recovery are intense and full of new emotions and wonder and hope.

> I was broke, my stomach hurt, I had a cloud of dread for the future, I dragged a chain of social shame around with me, but, boy, did I feel great.

I think some of us relapse because we want all of that feeling again.

Our minds steer us toward a relapse so we can start over. If going through the first six months was awesome the first time, wait until the second time; it will be even more awesome because this time I really know what I'm doing! We chase after that pink cloud the same way we chased after the first high.

In my first days of recovery, I had more free time than at any other time in my adult life. It was easy to get to a lot of meetings. There was always the hanging out after or before option. I was broke, my stomach hurt, I had a cloud of dread for the future, I dragged a chain of social shame around with me, but, boy, did I feel great. Any tiny little thing that happened to me that was in the least bit good was a true victory in my book. I drank a lot of coffee, ate a lot of donuts, and made a whole new group of friends.

As we get our shit together, there's less time to do all these things. I began working a second job. I picked up more freelance work. I started writing and submitting for publication. I went out more to perform and watch other performers. I started dating again. All of these things I wanted for myself, but they all required time from each day.

The revelations of self, instead of being enlightening, are obnoxious. At first when I saw that most of my problems in life were due to my bitterness, envy, jealousy, and sense of entitlement, I thought I would stop acting on those defects. I thought I would be magically rid of them once I hit my Seventh Step. But as that step says, we humbly ask to have these defects removed. It doesn't say that

> **As I saw my defects raise their heads from the lake of my character like the Loch Ness Monster, I'd always get bummed at another sighting.**

we get what we want. As I saw my defects raise their heads from the lake of my character like the Loch Ness Monster, I'd always get bummed at another sighting.

Our first friends that we made in recovery are not going to meetings anymore for one reason or another: a geographic reason, or their schedule doesn't allow it anymore, or they've relapsed. People move away for a job or to go back to school. Time gets sucked up in work, relationships, and child raising. Unfortunately, a lot of people don't stick with it.

I think what we all need is a second pink cloud where we feel joy and hope and see how far we've come.

## Finding Your Second Pink Cloud

There is definitely a second pink cloud to find. It's not in a relapse. You won't find it there. I doubt that's worked out for anyone, ever. Where should you look? I have three ideas on this.

### Pink Cloud by Proxy

I make it a point to spend social time with others who have less than a year sober. They're not my sponsees, but I watch them as they go through the steps. It's really exciting to watch people go from twitchy and depressed to healthy and happy.

To do this, I make sure to greet all of the people in my home-group. I'm not the official greeter, but I talk to each and every one of them. I at least introduce myself.

Years ago, during a pink cloud era, I always went out to eat with my homegroup after the meeting. We went en masse to a little burger place about half an hour before they closed and gave them more business than they'd had in the previous two hours. It was an awesome weekly party.

> **My pink cloud is hope, enthusiasm, and joy.**

But then we had to leave our meeting place at the same time the burger place cut its hours. Not only were we far away from the place at that point, but it closed an hour earlier, making it impossible to get there before closing time after the meeting. Then the usual attrition from the meeting happened: some quit coming, others had commitments to get back to after the meeting.

For a while, it was just me and one other guy. It was a letdown to not have the whole crew, but he and I got to spend a lot of quality time together. He was someone I'd met in a bar years before, and, like me, there was no doubt he needed to be in a program.

I got an idea one week that I should invite people individually, the same way I greeted them individually. So I went around after a meeting, checking in with the new people mostly, inviting them out with me to eat. My old method was to announce it before the close of the meeting or

> **Really understanding how far I've come in life and how everything has worked out for the better is a paddle shock to my wonder and amazement at the program.**

yell out, "who wants to go eat?" while the chairs were being picked up. Those are the ways that worked for me, but not everyone else thinks like me. Asking people individually worked.

Now, we have a crew of six regulars, but we end up with eight or nine every week. What's really awesome for me is that I'm spending more time personally with people who have less than a year in the program and who are not my sponsees. I hear about changes in their lives, the small revelations they have about themselves. I hear their troubles as they find jobs and start dating. The joy and excitement they feel, I can feel.

It really reminds me of the life that's been given back to me. Every moment I experience after Feb 19, 2002, is a second chance, a do-over, a mulligan. Really understanding how far I've come in life and how everything has worked out for the better is a paddle shock to my wonder and amazement at the program. My pink cloud is hope, enthusiasm, and joy.

This is a pink cloud by proxy. When I remember the benefits and the victories of the program by seeing them in other people, the little things in life that annoy me fade away. It's easy to get caught up in the tedious parts of life. It's easy to forget how far I've come and how awesome where I am now would have looked to me then. By socializing with a lot of short timers, I'm able to see my blessings through their eyes.

## Make Time for Your Pink Cloud

I've gotten so caught up in making up for lost time that I don't always take time off just to enjoy myself. I spent an amazing amount of time in bars sitting on a stool waiting for something to happen, and it never did. Then I got my shit together and starting doing things again. Then I got wrapped up in everything that I was doing.

The drunk life, the drug life, is a life of talk and ideas but little action. For years I complained about things I wanted to do but never did. While wasted, I came up with brilliant ideas that I never acted on. I made shit lists of people to blame for my failures and golden roll calls of the people who were on my side. I took notes on napkins. I called my answering machine to leave messages for myself to remember to do some genius thing that was unintelligible when I listened to it later.

As soon as I had a grasp on sobriety, I began chasing down old ideas. I was supposed to be a writer, damn it, and I hadn't had a book out or a manuscript together in years! There were plays to be in. Poetry readings to attend. I never finished school; I should go back and do that.

As I pursued my goals, I quickly ran out of time. The good side of this was that there was absolutely no time at all to get wasted anymore. How I'd ever found an entire day just to drop acid and recover from it astounded me. Multi-day speed binges would take a well-planned vacation to achieve now. The bad side was that I'd lost time for my favorite parts of sobriety.

It's really not hard to hit a meeting a day when you have nothing to do. Two meetings isn't hard if you live in the right cities. San Francisco has meetings on and off throughout the day in the same buildings, with libraries and cafes nearby to hang out in between. But as jobs and relationships and hobbies pop up, it's not so easy.

When I look back on my favorite moments in sobriety, copious free time always factors in. Killing hours between two meetings with another recovering addict. Rides to and from meetings. Hanging out with others after a meeting.

I'm not going to have that kind of free time again. Yet I do have time. I have to make time. I can get so caught up in this idea of making up for lost time, that I don't spend my available time the way I should have spent my time all along.

## Don't Forget to Enjoy Yourself

Sometimes I feel guilty for having fun. I feel that I should be doing something productive. That I should be at home writing the next book. That I'm spending too much money doing what I'm doing. I question positive feelings. They can't be good, can they?

My fun meter is damaged from years of drug use. What is fun? How do people have fun?

I had some fun times on drugs, so much fun I ruined years of my life trying to have that fun again. But what did I really think was fun back then about coke binges and all day whiskey drinking? What did I really enjoy about dropping acid at a music festival?

For me it was the people I was with. I felt like they liked me. I never felt comfortable socially unless I was drinking or getting high with others. All the social bullshit fell away.

> **There are game nights. Road trips. Vacations. Hiking. Camping. You need to find what you really enjoy to find your new pink cloud.**

Taking time to spend with others in sobriety is the key to my second pink cloud. Assuaging my inept social sense was what brought me happiness through drugs and alcohol, and it's what will work in sobriety.

It's sick but necessary for me to schedule time with my friends. I'll get wrapped up in work and not hang out with people. I'll listen to my isolationist voice that says I don't have anyone to hang out with. I'll come home and get lost in the DVR or the latest Netflix stash.

Every Wednesday, I rent out a theater and perform standup comedy with three of my friends. It's something that I never think I will have time for, but by the time I hit the stage, I think it's the best idea I've ever had. I'm tired after my day job and want to go home, or I have a writing deadline and think I should be writing, but as I get off the stage, I'm sure I did the right thing.

For you, I don't know what it would be. Some friends of mine surf. Others ride bikes. There are game nights. Road trips. Vacations. Hiking. Camping. You need to find what you really enjoy to find your new pink cloud.

# CHAPTER 5

# SITUATIONAL HABITS

**Once, one of my** normal friends asked me what people do after the Twelfth Step. "Relapse?" I said with a shrug.

I didn't know at the time. I was still wrapping my mind around the higher power concept back then. The idea of the Twelfth Step was so far off from me theoretically, I couldn't deal with it. I was still trying to understand how I was going to work through Step Two.

So I asked around. I heard the Thirteenth Step joke quite a few times. The Thirteenth Step, for those of you who don't know, is to fuck someone you met at a meeting. After the joke, I kept hearing the word "service." People found stuff to do, according to their talents, that kept them busy. Some had a herd of sponsees. Some secretaried meetings. Some did work with hospitals and institutions. That made perfect sense.

I became fascinated with people's relapses. What makes someone go out after a day, two weeks, a year, or ten years? Are we always really that close to a relapse? Don't we get any better? Frankly, it freaked me out. There were people who seemed totally on fire with the spirit of recovery one week who would show up the next week, raising a hand as a newcomer.

There are definite steps to recovery and sobriety, but what kind of steps lead us to a relapse? Is it just one? Using or drinking? Is it that one random Fuck-It action that comes up in our brains? One moment we're fine, and the next moment, we're making up for lost time in our disease?

There have to be steps that we're using to get to that point when picking up our old habits makes sense.

I spent the last Christmas I was drinking alone in a hotel room in Baltimore. I had all the whiskey I could handle and a couple of Cokes and an ice machine down the hall. There was a TV. I also had a burning resentment to keep me warm all night. Pretty much a perfect spirit of Christmas, if you had asked me at the time.

Just this past Christmas, because there was a full house at my dad's place, I stayed at a Super 8 Motel. Immediately upon entering the room, I had an allergic reaction to something in there, a reaction that was much like an asthma attack. I had to have some Benadryl; there was no other way for me to proceed.

> **There are definite steps to recovery and sobriety, but what kind of steps lead us to a relapse?**

There was one place still open, a gas station that also sold liquor. I picked out the allergy meds and looked right across the counter to the rack behind, full of whiskey, vodka, and rum. There was a fountain soda machine to the right. It would be easy.

That man would sell the whiskey to me if I asked for it. He wouldn't hesitate one bit. No one at the motel would think anything of it. There was no social stigma to face.

As quickly as these thoughts passed through my mind, I wondered why they had. Why do I feel a pull sometimes and not others? What makes a neighbor's cocktail on an airplane so much more tempting than seeing the same cocktail in a nightclub? When do I still want a drink?

It really didn't seem like eight years had passed for me between those two Christmases. They seemed only moments apart. The part of my brain that says Hotel Room Christmas equates it with Get Bottle of Whiskey. Then it made more sense to me. I hadn't spent a holiday

> **As far as I can see, the only solution is to power through it, and then you'll have a neural pathway that equates the situation with sobriety instead of drunkenness.**

in a hotel room sober before. It was in the list in my brain. It was a situational habit.

In my sober time, I had faced the same situations many times. Being in the comedy club, being at an art opening, seeing a wine list at a restaurant: I had seen all these moments often. I had experienced them sober hundreds of times. None of them was an issue anymore.

Just like a certain smell can bring you back to a specific moment in your life, a moment you may not have thought about in years or previously remembered, recreating a situation can take us back to a time of our drinking and using.

There's no way to avoid these situations, really. These random configurations of events, emotions, time, and place are too hard to reconstruct or notice beforehand. As far as I can see, the only solution is to power through it, and then you'll have a neural pathway that equates the situation with sobriety instead of drunkenness.

> **Just like a certain smell can bring you back to a specific moment in your life, a moment you may not have thought about in years or previously remembered, recreating a situation can take us back to a time of our drinking and using.**

### JEFF H.

Jeff H. is a 34-year-old bartender in San Francisco. In the little more than a year I've known him, I've watched him resolutely work his steps, do service, and work with others. Sometimes I see guys like him who really want the recovery. It kicks me in the ass a little, reminds me that the work never ends. Jeff is a solid guy.

Bartending is not an unusual job for a recovering alcoholic. In theory, it sounds like a contradiction, but the reality of it makes sense. Many people who have a bartender's access to alcohol end up with a drinking problem. Of those, some choose to quit. Most people don't have the luxury of quitting their job once they get sober. I have a soft spot for bartenders in recovery, since it was a sober bartender who took me to my first meeting.

"The first five years of bartending were exciting, glamorous, and fun," he told me. "I really thought I had become something. Then the next five years I loathed what I had become. I used to go to work and it took a drink just to set up the bar."

. Jeff has been clean and sober for one year and three months. Since he decided to join a program, he hasn't relapsed. "At first I tried to quit on my own," he told me. "I gave myself a timeline. I thought after a given amount of time I could drink like a normal person." That didn't work out for him.

"When I went into the program, I was done. My sponsor was lucky as shit when he got me. I was ready to do anything he said, show up on time, do the work.

"For the first year of my sobriety, bartending was my only job and I was just making it by financially. I had to stay sober to survive. Money-wise, I couldn't stop bartending. But then I saw how fucked up people get, how intoxicated they become. I see through their façade. I don't see it as people having a good time all the time. I see those like me, who on many nights take one shot too many and go over to the other side, the people with a thousand-yard stare; they're not enjoying it, they're just getting consumed by it.

"Alcohol has kicked my ass so hard. I know the full consequences of my drinking. Now, I can go home after work and wake up the next day without the feeling of hopelessness and despair, and I'll have money in my pocket.

"Coming to a 12-Step program brought me back to the feeling of doing a good job, having fun, and getting excited about doing it again.

"I try to squeeze in a meeting before my shift. If something happens at work, the next day the first thing I do is find a meeting. I also am in the habit of doing a Tenth Step with my sponsor on the way home. I'll leave it on his voicemail if I have to.

"On those days I don't feel like I have any negative things to unload, I'll list three things I did right that day. A Tenth Step isn't always about the bad things in our inventory."

## ETHEL PANCAKE

I met Ethel on the East Coast when I had four months sober. Like a dumbass, I thought it would be a great idea to go on tour newly sober. At four months, the longest I'd ever been sober since I started, I felt like I was solid enough to hit the road.

It was a spoken word tour for me, opening up for a queer hip-hop group. Touring was what I had missed more than anything. For years I was unable to get my shit together enough to go on tour. For one, there's the planning. Tours take an enormous amount of energy to set up. I never got past that. Had I gotten past that, I would have had to save money to pay for it. Most tours lose money, and you have to be ready to cover the entire cost yourself. There was no way I was saving money. So the offer to be the opening act was irresistible, even if the genre wasn't my scene and I was much older than the band members.

One night, two of my tour members decided to come back to the room where I was sleeping and smoke crack. Like, an ice tray full of crack. A lot of crack. I moved to a different part of the house, but the smell lingered in that room as well, that burning plastic army man smell. The tour people were the ones who never had any money, but they had a quarry full of crack. I figured they were into our tour money. I waited until they ran out and were coming down the next day. Then I let them have it. I reamed them. I made one of them cry and hide in the bathroom. I was riding high on righteous indignation to a level I have not experienced since.

I was told I might have to leave the tour, as yelling was not acceptable. To this day, I still don't understand why the crack was tolerated. That was never explained to me. Crackheads around our gas cash was fine, but anger was not. The person who owned the house? Crackhead. That's why. Although claiming to be just a casual crack smoker. Smokes crack like normal people. The logic that only makes sense to crack smokers.

I went to the gig that night not knowing where I would stay, when who did I run into but my ex-girlfriend, Myrtle. Ever the one for caring for the bird with the broken wing, the giraffe with the sore neck, and the newly sober suffering, Myrtle took to me right away. Wouldn't you know it, her girlfriend was a 12-Stepper working three different programs. That was how I met Ethel.

Ethel took me to a meeting the next day and later let me ramble on and on. I had never been so glad to get to a meeting. That was the first time I really needed another member to reach out and get me to a meeting or I wouldn't make it. I was freaking out, out of town, and Ethel was there for me.

Ethel has over ten years now, but she took a while to really get a clean and sober groove going. Her take on relapsing was, for her, age and a mindset coordinating with a whim.

"I'd stay sober for two years, then go out again. You decide you're going to do that and you do it. I think it's easier to do it when you're younger; you're so stupid when you're younger."

Now, however, she's resolved not to relapse, as she's well aware of the consequences of her actions.

"I hope I never have to drink again. I didn't feel it before; I hit bottoms; I went to a mental hospital; I was arrested."

I asked her what makes her susceptible to a relapse. Is it what you do, or what you don't do?

"If I get far enough away from the program . . . that includes step work and service, not only meetings . . . relapse is inevitable. I don't have an obsession, a craving, but I'm so crazy with resentment I could easily imagine not going to meetings, getting the Fuck-Its.

"Currently, I'm stacking cat food at a grocery store. There is alcohol in the store, but I don't have to work around it. I hardly see it. I do see my coworkers getting a six-pack to take home after work, and I'm ringing up my pint of ice cream. I really turned to ice cream as a reward for a hard day's work, for a while.

"I used to work these waitress jobs, and the thing was to take your tips to the bar after work. I want a treat after a tough day. It's not alcohol anymore. It's now ice cream.

"I did have a moment one day, a real moment after I mopped the floor where it seemed like the next thing to do was to go get drunk. After eight years of sobriety at the time. Some part of my subconscious equates hard work with drinking."

When I asked her how she's changed in sobriety, the topic turned to dating.

"I'm a lot less promiscuous now. That goes hand in hand with alcohol. And the dates themselves are much more creative. I like taking little trips. Going out of town to a sleazy motel. I never would have gone that far when I was drinking."

# CHAPTER 6

# AS LONG AS YOU HAVE
# IT ALL FIGURED OUT

**I was walking down** Market Street, headed to a meeting. This kid, early twenties, hits me up.

"Spare change for beer?" he asked.

"Fuck, no," I said.

I walked on. Then I stopped. I used to be like that kid. I'm no better than him, just at a different point in my life. I should try to help, I thought. I walked back.

"Hey, dude," I said. "Look, I'm going to a 12-Step meeting right now. It's right down the street. Like two blocks from here. You don't have to do anything, just come and have some coffee and hang out."

"No, that's okay," he said. "I'm not an alcoholic."

"Come on, my man," I said. "You're out here, hitting strangers up for beer money."

"It's not alcohol that's my problem. I'm more into narcotics."

I reasoned with him a little more, but it didn't do any good. He had it all figured out, much the way I had it figured out for years while friends, family, random strangers, medical professionals, bouncers, and police officers told me I had an alcohol problem.

Alcohol wasn't my problem. "The way the world is was my problem. Everyone is so fucked up out there, all fake and shit. Working jobs so they can afford a nice house and a nice car so they can show off to other people that they have nice things that they, deep down, don't even want; they just want to show that they're better off than the next guy. They're the ones with the problem. Why don't you tell them to sell the house and the car and quit working, huh? I'll tell you why you won't; because you've bought into it. They've already gotten to you."

Yeah, I had it figured out. You weren't going to catch me with a nice car and a nice house. Fuck that.

But what I do admire about myself in those days was the sheer resolution, the determination to get drunk, to stay drunk, and to drink some more. Nothing was going to stop me. The last way you would find me was sober.

My life was figured out. I knew what I was doing with the rest of my life, because the rest of my life was only until I lost consciousness, and that could be done relatively quickly. I never worried about what would happen any other day.

Live in the moment. Be in the now. Carpe diem. All that stuff, those ideas, I used in the worst possible ways. While they're supposed to be used for some kind of spiritual enlightenment, I was using them to reinforce my lack of consequence for my actions. Don't worry about the rent money, don't worry about the feelings of others, don't worry about your coworkers. I did what I wanted to do at the moment. My big goal was to complete my obligations for the day and drink until I woke up in the next day.

Newly sober, I tried to map out my life plan. I set goals for myself and accomplished them. I went back to school and got my BA, and I got a better job. But not everything worked out, and not on the schedule I wanted it to. I went through breakups. In finding that better job, I went through a series of rejections, not even getting interviews for many positions, to the point that I had given up on the process and decided to go to grad school, when the job showed up suddenly.

I thought I had it figured out when I was out drinking, and I thought I had it figured out newly sober. Now I've let go of the whole concept of having it figured out, which I think is a vestige of my drunken life. I don't have it figured out, and I don't think I can figure it out. It's life. It's much bigger than I am, and it will happen without me.

> I don't have it figured out, and I don't think I can figure it out. It's life. It's much bigger than I am, and it will happen without me.

Just like it says in the Serenity Prayer, knowing the difference between what we have control over and what we don't is true wisdom. That's all there is to figure out: what's yours to change and what you need to accept.

## Hold Fast

Sailors used to tattoo the words *hold fast* on their fingers right below the knuckles. The superstition was that the ink would keep them from going overboard in a storm. They would be able to hold on to the rigging. I like this imagery. No matter what storm comes up for you in your life, you can hold fast to keep from relapsing.

There are a lot of problems that you will face in your recovery that you have never faced without the influence of drugs. There were times that I loved bad things happening to me because they made it socially acceptable to get drunk. No one begrudges someone who gets drunk after a friend dies or after a big breakup. Getting wasted after bad news is the easy way out.

It's also easy to make excuses that inevitably blow up in our faces. The glass of champagne at the wedding or on New Year's Eve seems really innocuous to many, but to us, it's the crack in the dam. Calming the nerves before a flight, being at a convention where business is conducted over drinks, or being in a foreign country where people don't know what alcoholism really is can all be dangerous places for us. We can make trouble for ourselves quickly by bargaining a relapse or by making an exception to our rule.

> **No matter what storm comes up for you in your life, you can hold fast to keep from relapsing.**

We should have gradually built up an emotional skill set that would deal with our problems, fears, and anxieties. In our teenage years, we faced the smaller versions of life problems that we should've learned from. But while we were using and drinking to get through those hard times, we didn't build up any long-term abilities to deal with these situations.

Instead, we became callused to situations that should scare us. Scoring drugs, committing crimes to support our habits, and hanging out in seedy bars should frighten us, but it's where we're most comfortable. We know how to handle ourselves in a bar fight, but not at the office Christmas party. We would rather go Dumpster diving than to a dinner party. We're fine moving into a squat, but not getting an apartment with our partners.

> **I'm frightened of job interviews, the dentist, and first dates. I'm not afraid of drinking to a blackout, getting drugs from people I don't know, and letting drunks drive me home.**

I like to think of it as having a "fear detector" that's installed backwards.

I'm frightened of job interviews, the dentist, and first dates. I'm not afraid of drinking to a blackout, getting drugs from people I don't know, and letting drunks drive me home. I've risked my health, my freedom, and my relationships because I wanted to drink and use, but I was wary of doing many things that would improve my life.

The experiences we should have dealt with in our young lives we got through with the help of drugs and alcohol. Don't like your class? Get stoned before going. Nervous before a date? Have a few drinks first. All the times we had to face a responsibility or a fear, instead of building an emotional skill set to deal with it, we took the getting high shortcut.

Now we're facing a grownup life with a pubescent emotional skill set. Any emotion that we yoked together with drugs and alcohol is stunted. We need to exercise these emotions and strengthen them. Society at large expects us to be able to act our age. They don't know we may be fourteen inside.

## BARNABY

There's no way Barnaby goes unnoticed when he enters a room. He's a big man, big in body, energy, and spirit. He's covered in tats. When I met him, he was well over 300 pounds but lost 100 pounds on a bet. Still, his presence is as large as his appetite.

When I say appetite, I mean for everything, not just food. Barnaby likes what he likes a lot. He consumes. At times it was vodka, cocaine, or sex. It was and has been tattoos. They sprout from the cuffs of the hoodie and turtlenick he's wearing, their colors and designs up to his ears. He's owned more cars and bikes already than I will in my entire life. Don't get me wrong; he also loves food.

Barnaby is an easy man to talk to, despite all his leanings toward the rough, the scary, and all things scumbagish. If I described his tattoos or his Harley you may not picture the right man. Barnaby is one of the first strangers I talked to at a 12-Step meeting.

He's loud, he laughs freely, and he'll talk to anyone. The men's meeting that is my homegroup is dear to me in a big way because of him. At a time when I felt invisible in the rooms, I ran into him at the gym and he asked me why I hadn't been to the meeting more often. It was the first time I felt like my presence was missed.

Barnaby owns and runs a tattoo shop in a San Francisco neighborhood that is equal parts tourist and crusty punk. Looking out the front door, you're as likely to see a woman in Juicy Couture sweatpants shopping for shoes as you are a young runaway with tribal cat whiskers tattooed on his face. It's a street as contradictory as Barnaby's personality and his image.

I caught up with Barnaby at my favorite recovery-friendly restaurant, the Lucky Penny. Barnaby ate like he was trying to send all the foods in the kitchen a message, like he was trying to threaten them that they would be next. We talked about his business, and his monster breakup that was a sure trial for him spiritually and emotionally.

"Some people say, 'If you drink, you'll die.' Some people drink and die quickly. Some don't. When I say you aim at the ground, you're drinking as hard as you can. You are going to lose your job because you're drinking openly on the floor of your job, getting caught passing out at work, or coming out of a blackout at work; only an alcoholic does that. That's one of the ways to prove you're an alkie. If you're going to drink, you're going to drink like an asshole. We have the saying, 'Our hats are off to you if you can drink like a gentleman.' My hat is off to you if you can drink like an asshole and not have to come back. I don't want to drink like a gentleman. Gentlemen are pussies. I want to drink like an unmitigated shithead."

On his breakup:

"I knew what to do. I did another Fourth Step. My sponsor was on vacation in Mexico, so he told me, 'Get another sponsor you can talk to *now*.' I'm calling everyone in the group all the time.

"I'm running into my ex everywhere, on dates with guys I know. I'm getting in fights, and I move out of the city. But I did another series of amends; the IRS audit was the final amends.

"I went to 180 or 200 meetings straight. I did everything that was suggested. If you and sobriety had a good relationship, I'd listen to you. You know? I didn't drink. I'm still stupid enough to do stupid stuff. If you've done it two or three times drunk, you'll try it sober. Maybe not the same way. But if you're a car thief, and you get sober, now you're a sober car thief."

On working in an industry that caters to the user and drinker:

"Being a shop owner, I have a bit of control. I can choose not to hire people that I know are active users. No one who works for me is an out and out junkie. Two of my employees like to party, but they don't bring it to work. If you worked for Starbucks, you'd get fired. I know that it's an industry of the dysfunctional in a culture of the dysfunctional. I know a lot of tattoo artists have played with 12-Step groups, 1-2-3 out. Quite common with people I know. 'I got my meth under control so I can smoke pot and drink and not feel bad about it.'

"In my first few years, it was really confusing not drinking. It's really hard when I hang out with super famous tattoo artists who want me to do drugs with them. When I went to Japan, everyone drinks and expects you to drink with them, and if you don't drink, it's a sign of disrespect.

"I tell them it's my religion. My spiritual practice doesn't allow me to drink. They don't understand alcoholism culturally. There is 12-Step in Japan, but it's a white guy thing. There's drug problems. I heard a rumor that the yakuza own the rehabs as well as the drug distribution. They get their money on both ends.

"I have a friend who is a real drug dealer. Doesn't do drugs, doesn't drink, but the fact of the matter is, hanging out with him makes me itchy. If sobriety is my beautiful girlfriend, why would I hang out with a slut who wants to fuck me right now? I broke up with drugs and alcohol. But like a crazy ex who never stops calling, coke and booze never take no for an answer; they'll accept rejection, and they'll come around again. 'Sweetheart, I'll blow you in the back of the car; no one will know.'

"There's a lot of networking that happens inside of strip clubs and bars, and a lot of heavy hitters who like to party really hard. You have to say no; you have to leave. Maybe I'm not as much fun as I was when I was high. But I can have fun sober."

Here are Barnaby's tips on staying clean and sober at conventions:

> **If you have a reason to be there, fine. If you don't, leave.** When it comes to places that serve alcohol, Barnaby goes if there's a group going and networking to be done; he leaves once he's accomplished these things.
>
> **Have a sober wingman.** Who's your sober buddy? Barnaby's in favor of the buddy system the same way kids have buddies on school field trips.
>
> **Keep your phone numbers handy.** With a cell phone, there's no excuse not to call people if you start feeling a little weird.

# CHAPTER 7

# THE GREAT NOTME: ATHEISM, HIGHER POWERS, AND PRAYER

**Since writing *Get Up,*** the most asked question I get is how an atheist should deal with the higher power problem. Coming to terms with a higher power of your own understanding is the biggest hurdle the atheist will have in a 12-Step program. Those from conventional religion seem to have little to no problem assimilating their own beliefs to the steps and principles of the program. But entering any meeting, there's a proliferation of the word *god* everywhere, and most meetings I've been to have been in churches. What are we atheists supposed to think is meant by the word? Sure, we hear the phrase "higher power of your own understanding" but we also hear "god" many more times than that.

Being an atheist in recovery is only a problem in the short term. It was my biggest hurdle to get over initially, but now I look at it as an asset rather than a problem. In the long run, it helps me take the program's principles at face value rather than conforming them to a predetermined set of spiritual beliefs. After you figure out the nature of your higher power, there's no longer a conflict with your personal beliefs and your recovery. Let's look at the core of what atheism is all about.

Atheism, in its most basic form, is the lack of belief in a deity. That's it. There are as many different interpretations of this as there are of the Bible. Some atheists believe in an afterlife; some don't. Some believe in a supernatural power that's not deistic, like a mass consciousness, or a life energy. Atheism doesn't conflict with the idea that there is a power greater than yourself.

I don't believe in an anthropomorphic being that looks over me. I don't believe it's doling out experiences for me or has made a life plan for me. I don't believe it's watching out for me or making things happen. But I do believe in a power infinitely greater than myself.

I see my nonphysical self as a series of choices. I have decisions to make in this life, and those are in my control. Everything else in this big universe is my overall higher power.

There is an infinite number of things beyond my control. Relatively, there's not much that is in my control. Thus, everything that is beyond my control is a power greater than myself.

I call it NotMe. There's me and NotMe. NotMe is a higher power. It's not a deity, or a spirit, or even a vague concept. It's more of a negative space of everything that's not within my control. It's a higher power that should suit every atheist.

It fits really well with the Serenity Prayer and with the other instances of the word *god* as well. Dividing your life between what is yours and what is NotMe is what the Serenity Prayer is all about.

What I really like about NotMe is how it works said aloud. When someone's pissing me off, I say to myself "that's NotMe."

Maybe you'll like NotMine better. It doesn't matter what you call it, as long as you understand how it separates.

## Prayer and Atheists

I pray the same way I would talk to a car or yell at a sports team on television. It's not that I think they can really hear me, but it makes me feel better. In this sense, when I yell at a pair of dice to roll a certain number when I'm playing a game, I'm praying for a good roll although I know objectively that I can't affect the outcome. Luck doesn't work that way.

Atheists should pray. It's good for you. Just because you're not praying to something that can hear you doesn't mean you shouldn't do it. What is the good of this? It's my opinion that prayer works not because of reception, but upon transmission.

> **Atheists should pray. It's good for you. Just because you're not praying to something that can hear you doesn't mean you shouldn't do it.**

There were times when I was a practicing Christian that I was sure my prayers were being answered. I took that as proof that I was right in my religious beliefs. Most religious people would agree with this. They pray; they get results. I'm not arguing with the results; I'm arguing with the explanation.

I'm not saying I know exactly how it works. All of these people with their different versions of God and other deities, and yet prayer works for all of them. Either every religion is right, or prayer somehow works no matter what you pray to. I think that by the act of praying we activate something in our minds that helps us with our hopes and desires.

So if I'm an atheist and don't believe in a deity, where does prayer fit into my life? As a 12 Stepper, I do a regular inventory of myself. I look at this: Where have I been self-seeking or afraid? How have I been treating other people? Then I make a prayer.

I write the prayer down on an index card and carry it with me. I usually have one in my wallet or my pocket. I put the words in my head in that track that, left unguarded, will repeat negative thoughts and replay painful events and conversations.

You know the track I'm talking about. It says, "I'm not good enough. I don't deserve this. There's no way I'm ever getting this job." Or it repeats a many-years-old incident, where I say different things, and there's a better outcome. Or it imagines a fight I might have and what I would say during it.

This part of the brain serviced a lot of nights getting drunk. It spoke freely through the influence of cocaine. It's paranoid, self-deprecating, and blames others. Maybe yours is slightly different, but you probably have one.

Put the prayer in this track. Any time you start to slip into that headspace, repeat the prayer to yourself.

For example, while writing this book I might write down:

- I will not let my fear of sounding stupid stop me.

- I will write out of a sense of helping others, not
  out of pride.

- I will not procrastinate. I will keep up with the schedule I have made for myself.

It looks simple. It is. It's also been remarkably effective. I've used this type of prayer before job interviews, before dates, and before social functions. It's really good for keeping my head straight.

It's a lot like replacing a song that's stuck in your head with a different song.

## SRB

SRB is someone that I lived parallel to for a long time. We had a lot of friends in common, but we never ended up hanging out until he got into the program. We heard of each other's drunken exploits. SRB was in many bands with friends of mine. His loves are music and Burning Man.

With my homegroup, Burning Man was a punch line. It was everything we didn't like about hipster culture. We were mosh-pit drunks, while Burning Man people were glowstick-raver pill-poppers. We carried our judgment from our drinking days over into our sobriety. So when Brad showed up and started talking about Burning Man, we let him have it. To us, Burning Man was a place where we never went even when we wanted the drugs.

SRB soon proved to be a solid brother. He's always willing to help anyone out, sponsors many people, is always of service, and does a lot of little things to help out, like talking to the lonely rambling phone callers, and giving rides to those who can't seem to take a bus to a meeting. One of my favorite things about his sobriety is that he carries a joy with him that he spreads around the meeting, whether you want it or not. SRB loves being sober and being part of the program. That attitude makes it much easier for me to feel the same way.

"I loved stumbling through Burning Man whacked out of my gourd on acid, ecstasy, ketamine, GHB, mushrooms, pot, nitrous, and whatever else I could stuff into my system. The sensory overload was phenomenal.

"When I returned from Burning Man back when I was using, I would be incredibly exhausted and burned out for at least two weeks afterwards. When I returned from my sober burn, I got a good night's sleep and went back to work two days later feeling just fine. The difference was truly night and day."

But what of the Burning Man experience clean and sober?

"I loved stumbling through Burning Man totally clear-eyed and clear-headed. The sensory overload was phenomenal. I also noticed a helluva lot more of what was going on.

"With about six months sober, I went to Burning Man. Someone offered me drugs within twenty minutes of my arrival. I politely declined. Out of the blue, a couple of days later, someone tipped a drink to my lips and I recoiled as if from a hot flame.

"There are 12-Step camps there; one is called Anonymous Village. They have multiple meetings each and every day, rain or no rain, sandstorm or no sandstorm. I went to at least one meeting a day and usually two; it was great to hear about what people's experiences were like out there on the wild and woolly playa; Burning Man, being a supremely creative society based on giving instead of taking, is full of synchronicities, coincidences, and just plain god moments of quite magical intersections and connections. There is a large clean and sober community there, and if we stay connected, we are all stronger. God has an inordinate fondness for gatherings of alcoholics.

"I read selected spiritual readings and prayed and meditated every morning. I'd kinda always wanted to be one of those people who spread out a prayer rug towards the rising sun each morning. I like that idea of, like, honoring the great spirit and the coming day.

"Turns out, my sponsor relapsed at Burning Man the next year. The later autopsy of his sobriety revealed that he hadn't been going to enough meetings and also had some things going on that he hadn't been talking about."

I turned the conversation to SRB's work as a musician.

"I spend a lot of time in bars and nightclubs and gigging at drunken private parties and weddings. I've found drugs on the premises, held them in my hand, and had no desire to do them.

"This is because I am in good shape before I go into these situations. I go to enough meetings each week. I pray and meditate daily. I spend time each day trying to help other alcoholics.

"I've been granted immunity from the desire or temptation to get loaded, no matter where I am. The source power of the universe can do anything, and it does, provided I do what I need to each day.

"Most of the time I just go to the event and have a good time, but because I enjoy meetings, I usually try to get to a local meeting between sound check and show time, and I always have my phone handy in case I need it. I talk to the universe a lot and ask it for guidance and direction. If a member calls me and I have a moment, I always spend time talking to them, to connect, check in, and remind us of what our focus needs to be and how to live in the solutions instead of the problem.

"I stopped smoking at two years sober. I did start playing online video games obsessively. Quitting smoking was much easier than I thought it would be. First off, I was ready to quit. At least a pack of cloves a day for seven years is not good for you, and it runs about $200 a month. When the addict mind said 'cigarette,' I treated it like it was the same voice that said 'drugs, booze,' and I saw it for what it was, an alcoholic/addiction thought, and let it pass, and it did. I also took that moment to turn it into a little prayer of gratitude, saying, 'thank you, for making me a nonsmoker.' I did this over and over and over again, as necessary throughout the days. It definitely got easier after the first few weeks. I probably went through more bubble gum and mints than usual in the beginning, but quitting smoking without all the patches and gum and stress is totally doable. The higher power can do anything.

"Totally over 'em now, no desire at any time. I'm a nonsmoker again, end of story, and I like it that way. I didn't get sober just to die of cancer.

Continuing our conversation about common sober vices, we turned from smoking to sex.

"I'm basically still a virgin in sobriety. After three years, I've had my chances and have passed them up. In those cases, they were relative newcomers, and that would be unethical. Addicts and alcoholics are people who are always looking for something external to makes us feel better, and once drugs and alcohol are no longer options, many of us switch to sex. After you've been sober long enough and worked some steps, you'll realize this.

"Not only is it taking advantage of people in their space, it's potentially fatal to their recovery. This disease can easily be life or death for some of us at the point where we come to the program, and you cannot interfere with people's right to recover by selfishly pursuing your own sexual agenda. Well, you *can*, but it makes you an asshole. Part of the reason I'm into this program is so that I don't have to be an asshole anymore.

"A lot of people say that relapse is a part of recovery, and that may be true for some people, but on another level it's kinda bullshit, a saying that the disease uses to convince the addict/alcoholic to feed it what it wants. I've heard many people say they've had that thought run through their heads before they relapsed, and it led them to say 'fuck it' and go get loaded. When I came in, they told me I didn't ever have to drink or use again. I said, 'Well, shit, I want that.'

"I don't want to be one of those guys who drifts in and out for years and years without really getting it. That meant that I had to do the things suggested and go to meetings. I hit around 600 my first year.

"I like being sober because I feel like I have the opportunity to achieve my destiny, as opposed to sliding down to meet my fate."

# CHAPTER 8

# NOT MY BUSINESS

**The scariest thing I've** done sober is a job interview. Our fear detectors are installed backwards. What should be exciting opportunities, for us are frightening realities. What scares normal people, we accept without fear, and what we are afraid of is harmless.

Most people would be afraid to go into certain neighborhoods, buy drugs from people they don't know, and then use those drugs with needles of questionable hygiene. Each step of that would terrify most people. It's a process most people will never experience. Yet addicts do it on a regular basis, as much as their fix dictates.

I worked for years trying to get a better job. I went back to school and finished my degree. I sent out stacks of résumés. I hit up everyone I knew to find work for me where they worked. Everything was cool until I got to the job interview.

Job interviews are rough for a lot of people. I have some fear that they'll find out I'm a big drunk and not want to have me work for them. Some interviewers ask why I bounced around from job to job in several different industries. It's a little weird that I didn't get my BA until I was 35. There's a lot of underachieving that I put up with. I don't know how to explain it other than I had a drinking problem that kept me from fulfilling commitments and living up to my full potential.

I looked for better employment for several years. I gave myself a deadline and if there wasn't a job lined up for me by that date, I'd just go back to school and get a master's degree. I gave myself an either/or, and I let it go. It was now NotMy problem (NotMy being my higher power for that moment). My problem was looking for who was hiring and sending out résumés. Whether I would be hired was NotMy problem.

I prayed for serenity to accept whether or not I would get hired, and the courage to look for work and go on interviews. I admitted I was powerless over whether I would get hired. I turned over the will to be hired to my higher power. I took an inventory of the jobs I'd had before. I took an inventory of what I wanted from my life on a financial level. I looked at what made me a good or bad employee in the past. I looked at how my defects of character affected what kind of job I wanted and what kind of financial level I wanted to attain. I worked a whole series of steps around that job and then just let it go.

Then I got a call for a really cool job. There was this one job with a university editing course materials. The job would be perfect for someone like me who has a little bit of knowledge in a whole lot of areas. Correcting the mistakes of others would also be a healthy outlet for my control issues.

Fear struck. I would have to go down there and interview. If they had told me to go down and fight the guy for the job, I would've been fine. I would've done it. I'm not afraid of getting whupped. That's been done to me plenty of times. What I was afraid of was honesty, answering this man's questions in an honest manner.

I was afraid of him judging my life's choices. I was afraid of him not thinking I was qualified for the job. I was afraid he'd think I was too old for the job. But luckily for me, I had a handy list of all that fear, and it was NotMy problem.

I went in to the interview. I let go of all my preconceptions and my will. There were two paths for me: job or grad school, and it was NotMy decision. I reminded myself to answer everything honestly and went in.

During the course of the interview, I received some new information: they were hiring ten people for that job title. Immediately a rush of feelings hit me about that. First, my self-esteem had to chime in, and say, "Hey, asshole, if you're not any better than eleventh best for the gig, you really don't deserve this job." Next, my paranoia kicked in with the thought, "Yeah, they'll hire ten people, but only keep the five they like, and the rest will be laid off." I told those voices to can it, and that we would all stick with the plan that it was NotMy decision. NotMy business.

> **Fear struck. I would have to go down there and interview. If they had told me to go down and fight the guy for the job, I would've been fine.**

Had they told me they were interviewing ten people and that we were going to fight it out, Battle Royale style, to see who got to stay, I'd be down. Why? Because I'm an idiot. Anyway, that's not how it went.

I got that dang job, and it set off a whole new set of problems. I had fears of being laid off without warning, which had happened to me in the Dot Com days. I had resentment over people fifteen years younger than me being able to have the same job and pay that I did. I retroactively resented every previous employer who hadn't paid me what I was worth. I had to face my fear of the dentist and the doctor once my health plan kicked in. Give us what we want, and we'll find reasons we like What Wasn't Good Enough better.

I really encourage you to make fear lists like this whenever something comes up. Even if you don't think it's worthy of being afraid over. If you have fears, then you should not ignore them. You should figure out what they are exactly and let go of them. Pray about them. Share about them. Call your sponsor. Call your other program buddies. Don't act like they're not real. They'll only get scarier.

## Tips for the Dreaded Job Interview

Don't tell them you're a drug addict. I tend to blurt it out in many social situations. This is a good time to keep your own business private.

Don't go in smelling like cigarettes. It's perfectly legal, but if you smell like you've been hotboxing in your car before going in, it makes a bad impression. We 12 Steppers are used to people who chain smoke, but most people are turned off by it.

Don't drink too much coffee beforehand. You want to be alert, but you shouldn't be fully tweaked out. Again, it's almost a joke to us when we drink too much coffee, but you don't want to come across this way.

Watch your mouth. Don't swear. It's hard. Nothing calms me down in a conversation like dropping a "motherfucker" or "sonsabitches" in there. But it's definitely not the time and place for it.

Be jovial but not a comedian. We have a sense of humor that the normies don't have. We find the dark, the self-deprecating, and the obscene funny. Your laughter will disturb others.

Don't insult your past employers. Don't talk about how they were a bunch of lame-ass motherfuckers. Don't look like you're carrying a resentment or holding a grudge against them.

Where do you picture yourself in five years? Don't make a smartass remark, like "rehab." Don't be too Zen either and say something like "five years older." Say you want to be a homeowner or be married or have a family or something. Something normal, for fuck's sake. Try to pass.

### ALEX

Alex is a 29-year-old case manager at a halfway house for female recovering addicts. She has six years sober.

"I'm an addict who, if it's addictive, will go with almost anything. I started going to meetings because cocaine and a few other things had taken over my life and I didn't want to be ruled by something else. Since I've gotten clean from coke and managed to put together something resembling a sane and healthy life, I've been working on making sure I don't just transfer my addiction to something else—food, work, sex, etc.

"I have not relapsed with coke, which I count myself incredibly lucky for. Every other person I used with or copped from is dead or in jail. I was pretty close to both those options when I quit. What kept me from picking up coke again is a bunch of things. I learned, after a couple years clean, that I have a heart condition that was possibly caused by my use, and any further use could literally make me drop dead. It's pretty sobering that it could all end like that. I also lost everything when I hit my bottom—my relationship, my job, my home—and I keep at the front that it could happen again, just like that. I also want more out of my life than I had when I was using. Today I make art and write and enjoy my life with all the bullshit that it contains. I can get through the bullshit now, whereas I got mired in it before.

"I work in the recovery field, which has its plusses and minuses. Being in recovery gives me a great outlook that some folks who aren't in recovery might not be able to have; sometimes it's easier for an addict to relate to another addict. However, the personal downside is unique for the field: it's hard to remain even semi-anonymous in my program, as I live in a medium-sized working class city where everyone knows everyone else, and I do not blend in well. I don't often feel like a part of the recovery community, as I work as a professional in the field, and it can be really lonely. It also feels that sometimes, when other people in recovery find out what I do for work, people think I have all the answers. This really couldn't be further from the truth.

"When you're in a position of authority, even just by having more time clean than someone else, it's easy to make that into a self-fulfilling prophecy and actually believe you have all the answers; that's where some real shit starts, in my experience. It's easy to build a resentment on that because I am just as sick and just as fucked up as anyone else. I just happen to get paid to sit across a desk and help someone else get to a place where they're maybe a little less sick or a little less fucked up. It's hard to be of service, too, when I'm helping addicts forty hours a week. I'm not necessarily motivated to talk to folks who need sponsors, or need to do commitments, or what have you.

"That being said, I go to meetings out of the area where I can actually be anonymous when I can. I make sure I do my recovery separate from my day job, that I'm taking time for me and my issues, not just the issues of others. I leave my job at my job; when I'm off, I'm *off.* I try to remain open to folks who need help at meetings, and I do sponsor when I'm asked. Sometimes the biggest part of not picking up is to be fucking honest. Cough up the emotions and talk to someone about how I'm hating my meetings this week, or I haven't been writing my step work because work is really killing my soul this week, or whatever. A real bonus for me with my work is that it's a constant reminder of where I can end up if I don't take care of my shit.

"I think sometimes a misconception about people who have stopped using is that we're no fun. I think I'm pretty fun, and I think my sober friends are pretty fun, so I think sometimes being an example that we are not all self-important windbags who sit in a church basement eight hours a day is important.

"My experience has also been that, regardless of whether you're an addict or you're normal, the principles of 12 Step can be helpful. Trouble at work? Do a Step One and a Step Four on it. Your boyfriend/girlfriend making you crazy? Step One the fuck out of it, and then do a Step Four and a Step Nine on it, too. The steps and tools are transformative and can be used in a variety of situations and can be used by normal people, too. They're fucked up, just in different ways than we are. Sometimes the gift of help extends outside the setting of a meeting.

"The word *powerless* in Step One pushed a feminist button. I was brought up to be a strong and independent woman, and to have to sit down and reconcile that there were areas where I was not powerful and could not stand alone fucked me up good for quite a while. The idea of not being able to be independent and fix my addiction on my own under my own steam and to admit that I wasn't strong and willpower wouldn't save me is hard. I still struggle with the concept of powerlessness. It's still a fight.

"The movie *Requiem for a Dream* terrified me and made me physically ill. I saw it not too long after I got clean, and it was a living nightmare for me. I had picked up dope only a few times, but it terrified me on a seriously primal level. I don't think I slept for a couple of days.

"Lots of the music I listened to before and after I got clean helped in ways I didn't really know. I only found out after I came out of the haze that a lot of my favorite punk bands were clean and sober and my attitude became 'Well, if those motherfuckers who I saw shitfaced at the Rat (or wherever) got it together and can still play and still live their lives, I certainly fucking can.' I never realized that there was a serious segment of punks who were clean and sober and who weren't straight edge.

"I think one thing that a lot of the books about recovery don't mention or omit is that relapse is a part of recovery. If it wasn't, there wouldn't be so much shit written about it and 12-Step meetings would be constant revolving doors. To essentially make a lifestyle change, literally overnight for some of us, is a big fucking deal; and for many of us, it doesn't always stick the first time. I think the largest issue with relapse that doesn't get addressed is not the actual act of picking up but the shame around it. I have never met a person who relapsed who woke up the next day and was totally fucking fine with themselves, and that sometimes keeps people from coming back.

"I also think that those of us who attend meetings can sometimes get stuck within our own self-imposed limits based on what we see as the rules of 12-Step meetings. I'm of the opinion that whatever works . . . works. Sometimes I think we forget that the only requirement for showing up at a meeting is that you want to stop whatever it is that you're doing. Beyond that, you can pick what works. Yeah, the steps are a good option, but if you're staying clean and working it without 'em, who the hell am I to say you're doing it wrong?"

## Thirteen Things Every Addict Should Stop Doing

Here's another list that will help you take yourself out of the process that you used to have when living the life. The further you take yourself out of your drug and alcohol persona, the better off you'll be. Some of these things are directly related to using, and some are only tangentially related. Either way, the more you separate yourself from these actions, the better off you'll be.

### Pissing in Bottles

This one's for the fellas. Ladies, take a break. Really, this is a leftover part of your junkie life. There's no reason for it anymore. Probably the best reason for doing it is because you can, and that's stupid as hell. I understand those times when you're so fucked up that you don't know if you can find the bathroom, or you're afraid you'll run into your roommates and they'll see how trashed you are. I remember being on acid one time and not understanding how to get out of my room. I knew it had something to do with the doorknob, but I couldn't make the connection.

> **The further you take yourself out of your drug and alcohol persona, the better off you'll be.**

### Table Surfing/Dumpster Diving

Table surfing is the art of running through a restaurant and yanking up all the unfinished food from the plates of diners who are done. It's a great skill if you're homeless. You will not go hungry in an urban area if you're good at this. People leave a lot of food on their plates. But now you should be able to fend for yourself. Leave the surf to someone else.

Dumpster diving goes along with table surfing. I know some skilled folks who have furnished apartments and made some really cool artwork out of discarded items. There are those, too, who are *freegans*: those who only eat and use what they get for free. I'll draw the line here: if you Dumpster dived to support your drug life, then don't do it anymore.

## Saving Lost Causes through Dating

This one's the hardest on those of us with one alcoholic parent. We go from being the drunk parent to the enabling parent. Neither one is healthy. We see men trying to save damsels in distress and women standing by their misunderstood men. Men have this drive to rescue, while women have the same drive to support. Men will find the strung out stripper or the addict selling herself for drugs or drug money, and women will enable the drunken mess and put up with his emotional and physical abuse. None of this is right, but it's how we've

> **Men will find the strung out stripper or the addict selling herself for drugs or drug money, and women will enable the drunken mess and put up with his emotional and physical abuse.**

seen adults act throughout our childhood. We become obsessed with this person as a way to replace our drinking and using obsession. We switch from using to enabling. The enabling is also debilitating.

## Drug Dealing

Seems obvious, but I've met quite a few people in recovery who keep dealing while trying to get sober. There are many who think they'll be better at it once they quit using. I do have a double standard in some way here. There are a lot of sober people working in the nightclubs and bars. I don't think it's being around the supply that's tempting as much as being around the lifestyle and the moral crises that arise in the drug world. While the alkie bartender has to see and smell the alcohol, he's not engaging in illegal activity; nor does he have to act in a way that's contrary to a clean and sober life, morally. You can't deal drugs without coming into contact with violence, theft, and emotional manipulation. If you're not doing it, someone else near you is. Someone's lying and stealing to get the money to score from you. You could make the same argument for alcohol in bars, but it's not the same.

> **Everyone makes mistakes in life, but you made yours in permanent ink. I'm not saying you have to stop getting tattoos, by no means. Just stop getting the bad ones.**

## Hustling

I'm counting this as any scam that's either not legal nor drug dealing. Hustling is any kind of scheming-type plan where you end up getting over by doing something off the books or taking advantage of someone else. Whether it's selling something at work without ringing it up, or selling something that "fell off the truck," it's still a part of your process that you use to score drugs.

## Homemade Tattoos

Really. Look at the ones you have. Compare the ones you got for free versus the ones you paid for. Or depending on your case, the ones you got for free versus the ones other people have that they paid for. The phrase "a cheap tattoo is a bad tattoo" is often true, and a free tattoo really looks like shit. We've gotten to a place in our society in which tattoos are somewhat acceptable. I work in a regular office at a university, and they have no problem with my tattoos that are showing. I'm glad they can't see them all. Don't get me wrong, I think there's something charming about homemade Black Flag tattoos or words with letters that grow smaller or bigger as it goes, but the rest of the world thinks they look stupid, and by default, you are less intelligent for having them. Everyone makes mistakes in life, but you made yours in permanent ink. I'm not saying you have to stop getting tattoos, by no means. Just stop getting the bad ones.

## Thug Life

If you live, look, and act like a criminal, society will treat you like one. What gets you respect in the clubs, bars, and drug scenes will get you suspicion in the normal world. People will doubt your moral character based on the way you dress, your posture, and your general attitude. This may not be fair, but it's the way it is. If you roll up to a place looking like you're going to rob it, they're not going to hire you for a job. Unless the job you're going for is an extra in a gangsta rap video, put on a shirt, and stop with that prison yard stare. Move your mouth when you talk, and don't accentuate sentences by punching your open palm. Don't tell stories about fights you've

> **If you roll up to a place looking like you're going to rob it, they're not going to hire you for a job.**

had or any crimes you've committed. People are paying attention; they're listening.

## Living in SRO Hotels

The SRO (single resident occupancy) hotels are there in case of an emergency or as a last resort. By any means, they should be considered a temporary solution. They should not be a way of life. The hotels contain more drug addicts than they contain working people who are down on their luck. You're that much closer to the lifestyle by living in one. I've been in many hotels where that smell of meth, crack, and cigarette smoke permanently scented the place right over the barf-and-ammonia smell. It's not like they're cheaper, either. In most cities, the SROs are a little more expensive than renting a studio apartment in the same neighborhood. The difference is they don't look for a credit check, and they come with furniture. Here's my solution for this problem: subletting.

I've been subletting most of my life in San Francisco. It's a lot cheaper than getting a place all to myself, and many people will take you at your word, since they're living in the same house with you. Definitely until my credit sorted out seven years into sobriety, there was no way I was going to pass a credit check. For the furniture problem, there are always people getting rid of furniture that you can get really cheap or free if they know you. Don't worry about it not matching. One piece at a time, get it together.

## Hookers and Strip Clubs

There are many addicts who never went to strip clubs or solicited prostitutes while using. Definitely, if they were a part of your story, you shouldn't go for obvious reasons. But people quit spending money on drugs and then suddenly, they can afford strip clubs and hookers. Compared to smoking crack or shooting dope, it looks pretty harmless. But there's a transference issue here. It's really easy for us as addicts to let vices such as these demoralize us and dominate our lives. Outside of discussing any public health risks or making moral judgments of these places and actions, it's dangerous to the addict's psyche to become a regular customer of such establishments. I look at strip clubs as if they were bars. Some people can go to bars and drink now and

> **Camping in a van is one thing. Camping every day under a streetlight in a VW minibus is another.**

then. I've realized that I can't. I always tried to get a little drunker than the last time. I was always in search of that perfect bar. I could easily do the same with the clubs.

### Living in a Van

Much like the SRO problem. Living in a van is for hippies from another era. Even hippies of today should not live in a van. Camping in a van is one thing. Camping every day under a streetlight in a VW minibus is another. The benefit of living in a van is simple: no rent payments. That frees up your money to be spent on crack. The problem with it is, once you get used to this downsized life, it's hard to go back for several reasons. It's hard to start paying rent again. Just the idea of it seems like robbery. To get an apartment, you need to give them a reference from the last place you lived, and if the reference is from too long ago, or you tell them you're living in your van, you're not getting the place. From a financial standpoint, you have to save up the first and last month and a security deposit. From van life, you've likely stopped saving money, although ironically you need very little to live.

## Payday Advances

These places are predatory lenders. Stop going there. It's not even legal in some states. Loan sharks have often charged less. I saw one that collected $15 interest for a two-week loan of $100. I was never around the street loan bookie thing very much, but I did hear one guy saying he charged two points, which on this loan of the same amount would be $4. Mind you, the bookie is charging 104% interest, give or take, and the payday advance place in this example is charging several thousand percent. Someone out there, do the math and email me. The point is that these places are ripping you off.

> **If you can't afford it, don't buy it. There are places to buy things cheap if you can't afford full retail.**

## Rent to Own

If you can't afford it, don't buy it. There are places to buy things cheap if you can't afford full retail. Thrift stores, Salvation Army, and Goodwill have the same furniture for much cheaper than what you'll pay over the long term if you rent it. If Craigslist.org serves your town, you can often find items for little or nothing. Then there's always asking around the other people in the program. A lot of us were given things to use when we were new, and we're glad to pass them on to others.

## *Cursing*

I would love nothing more than to converse only in George Carlin's "Seven Words You Can't Say on Television." Even as a well-read man, my favorite word is *fuck*. It's good as every part of speech in the vernacular. It can express a grand multitude of meanings and be used in all kinds of situations. It was, at times, the only word I could still say through a drug haze. In my opinion, it's the best word in the English language, for its versatility, simplicity, and understandability. Fuck is our aloha. If you're Hawaiian and you have both of those words at your disposal, I don't think you need any other words.

The problem with the word, however, is that it's not socially acceptable in a lot of situations. It offends a lot of people. Sometimes they stop listening to what you are saying because they are so shocked that it's falling easily out of your mouth. Believe it or not, some people never say the word, and when they have to quote it they either whisper it or mouth the word to the other person. People refer to it as "the f-bomb" and "the f-word" because they don't want to really use it.

> I would love nothing more than to converse only in George Carlin's "Seven Words You Can't Say on Television."

For those of us who have spent a lot of time in bars, around tweaked-out drug scenes, or have done time in a penal institution, we've lost the concept that it's anything but a superhero-style pronoun that can be used in the place of any other word that can't surface in our brains at the moment. Consider this conversation:

"Dude, how the fuck are ya?"

"Pretty fucking good, how 'bout yourself?"

"Fuckin' A. Can't complain."

"You'll never guess who the fuck I ran into the other fucking day. Oh, fuck me. I just lost his fucking name. Just fell right out of my fucking brain just now."

"Oh, I hate that fucking shit. I swear, I only killed the brain cells that remember people's names and where my fucking keys are."

Normal conversation, right? Wrong. That's normal for us. Not for the rest of the world. Amongst ourselves, fuck it. Say whatever the fuck you want. But in the rest of the world, watch your fucking mouth. Basically, don't ever say it to anyone you don't know personally that you run into in the course of your day, either face to face or on the phone.

Here are some prime people you should never say "fuck" around, and times when you should never utter the word:

• Policemen and other authority figures

• During job interviews

- While talking to customer service reps on the phone
- Retail staff employees
- Within earshot of people's children

# CHAPTER 9

# COFFEE, CIGARETTES, PORN, GAMBLING, AND FOOD

**These days if you** see a group of people standing outside a building smoking together, they're either in front of a bar or a 12-Step meeting. If they're holding little Styrofoam cups, they're drinking coffee, and they're 12 Steppers. The two last holdouts of smokers are those in bars and those in recovery.

Twelve Steppers smoke more than people in bars, and we drink more coffee than anyone. There are no other groups that drink coffee all hours of the night unless they are trying to stay up for work. We put cabbies and medical interns to shame. Air traffic controllers are less buzzed than we are on a Tuesday.

Smoking is addictive, and so is caffeine. There's also sugar, porn, and gambling. Video games, working out, and house cleaning. Where does it stop? Can we really get addicted to anything? It sure seems so.

But there isn't just one meaning of the word addiction. Being addicted to cigarettes is not the same as being addicted to crack, and every drug addict knows this. But both are extremely hard to quit.

I bring this up because I've heard people use the issue as a reason to keep using and drinking or as a general slam on the "hypocrisy" of recovery. People will say they don't want to get into a recovery group because they'll just pick something else up. This may very well be true. A lot of people do; we call it transference.

Transference happens when you quit doing one thing but end up being equally obsessed with another thing. A lot of drug addicts are immediately addicted to anything that gets them high the first time. They've already built that pathway in the brain that allows for nonstop self-pleasure. In the drug addict life, they may switch from pot to Vicodin to cocaine to heroin and be using at pro levels almost immediately.

Similarly, when we quit drugs and alcohol, we can easily turn our obsession from our old vices to new ones that we don't see as dangerous. Some of them aren't as dangerous, and some of them are. Some things we are addicted to ruin our lives, demoralize us, and hurt those around us. Less problematic are the ones that only give us cancer and kill us.

## The Addiction Scale

So how do we rate these addictions? I'm listing them in a scale for my purposes here. While I think that marijuana is addictive and has stolen away the ambitions of people I know, I don't think their fate is the same as someone who has to constantly score crack all day and night. At the top of the scale are the worst things to be addicted to, and at the bottom, some that are not so bad.

Let's put crack and heroin at the very top. I don't know which one is worse to be hooked on. Both of them will tear apart your existence until you exist only to use. Both of them will demoralize you quickly, so you will rationalize any behavior that helps you acquire and use more. Both of them are extremely difficult to quit.

I'm going to put the different street versions of speed below crack and heroin, but it's close behind, especially if it's shot instead of smoked or snorted. An IV speed user is well into a physical addiction. Tweakers can lose all sense of moral boundaries quickly. A tweaker looking to get high won't have any problem committing a crime to support his habit, but the sad irony of speed is that he'll come up with a horrible plan and not be able to execute it properly. The reason I put it beneath the other two is, from my experience, those who walk away from it have a lower relapse rate. There's something more consuming about crack and heroin. I think there's more hope for the speed addict than for those using crack or heroin, so it goes just beneath them on the list.

Right beneath that, I'll place cocaine and the prescription drugs. I separate crack and cocaine. If you haven't done them or been around both, you may not know the difference. But I'm sticking with this delineation. People who are using cocaine and drugs that aren't prescribed for them seem to keep some kind of functionality about their lives. Maybe they hold a job or still live with family members. Heroin and crack seem to take people onto the street more regularly and quickly.

Alcohol: cunning, baffling, and delicious, is level three. What makes it special is that the detox from alcohol is the most dangerous of all. It's the only potentially fatal detox. The addiction curve is slower than the others I've mentioned so far, but once the physical addiction kicks in, the body literally needs a drink like it needs food, air, and water. An alcoholic can die without it. However, some alcoholics can function while feeding their addiction for many years without hitting bottom.

The fourth level I want to split into two blocks: nicotine and marijuana. Physically, the pull from nicotine is so strong that even while in the hospital for respiratory problems, patients still demand to smoke. Most smokers want to quit on some level, but in reality, never will give it up. Quitters relapse often and are soon back to smoking their old amounts. Marijuana, while not involving the harsh physical pulls of nicotine in the user, has an equal emotional tie to the mind of the user. While I would not consider the vast majority of users to be addicts, the ones who are have their lives focused around using, often changing careers, relationships, and quality of life to accommodate their addictions.

On the fifth level, I'm putting coffee by itself. Coffee has physically addictive properties to the extent that drinkers who do not get their usual coffee will get a headache. Emotionally, the bond is strong. A coffee drinker will be loyal to a particular brand of coffee for years, if not a lifetime. And the more you drink, the more drinking more sounds like a great idea. The solution to too much coffee is more coffee.

On the sixth level are sugar, snack foods, and chocolate. These are all food items that people have a hard time not eating when they don't want to. They don't feel addictive at all until you try to go on a diet and stop thinking about candy bars, cookies, ice cream, and cheeseburgers. The mere idea of not eating something like this can drive a person to go to the store and get some. While no one is going to be homeless because they like French fries, eating these things does change the quality of life people want to lead.

There are three common nonconsumable addictions that I don't know where to put: sex (including porn), gambling, and online gambling. I would like to put them between the cracks of each of these other levels because they exist in wide grades. Someone who is addicted to internet porn is not risking the same as someone who is addicted to sex with prostitutes, yet they're both sex addictions. I want to include gambling because there is such a strong physiological rush involved that I have commonly heard addicts say that gambling was like sex, better than sex, or that it was their sex. These two addictions could be coming from the same part of the brain. Online gaming I'm throwing in here because I need to put it somewhere, and it's a bit like gambling with respect to the emotional and psychological connection with the user.

Why bother with all of this?

It's good to know that all these things are addictive. It's also good to be able to explain that to someone when they say that pot isn't addictive. To them, the word addiction may apply only to the first few categories. When some people think of addiction, they think of someone prostituting themselves in exchange for drugs or stealing for drug money. They may not think about losing the drive to do anything all day except watch TV and eat Pringles.

# BERNADETTE

Bernadette is one of my writer friends. We got sober within a year of each other. I've watched her writing deepen emotionally and her career explode since she got sober six years ago. We go back a long way, back to when I was still feeling out my career as a writer.

Back then, I was part of a whole scene of young writers, standing right outside of the boundaries of San Francisco's literary scene. There were old Beat-era poets, barroom Bukowski wannabes, and issue-laden performance artists. The city always had our heroes reading, people like Kathy Acker, Dennis Cooper, and Jack Micheline. If you liked a writer, chances are, he or she eventually would read in San Francisco.

The literary scene was rife with drugs and alcohol. It wasn't hard to find free drinks, and it didn't take much more work to get a free high. We got loaded and talked about books and how to get published, and we got tweaked out and went on writing binges.

What worked for me for a long time, however, worked against me later. I stopped editing and rewriting. I began to miss deadlines; then later, I stopped submitting altogether. Then I didn't even finish pieces anymore. The drugs and alcohol affected us in many different ways, but one thing was common: they were putting our careers in jeopardy. Some of us chose our careers; others chose the drugs.

Bernadette's email interview was so good, I did very little editing or commentary.

"I haven't relapsed. I get tempted sometimes if I am having a hard time emotionally, like if I get in an emotional fight, over romance usually. I get this giant flare of craving in my body. Usually

I just smoke a cigarette and it goes away! Really, even if I don't smoke, it goes away anyway. I know that all cravings pass (and all emotions pass, and all problems pass) and so I don't ever need to pick up. The reasons for wanting to drink will go away, unless I actually drink, and then all problems will multiply. Just thinking it through for even a second helps banish the craving. I really don't want to be trapped in the cycle of despair that drinking brings on.

"I'm a writer, and I wrote and performed a lot drunk and really leaned on drugs and alcohol to help me along. It worked for a while, and then it stopped, and it will never work again. It is a mental dead end for me to wish that I could have a drink and get lost in my writing or do a line and be funny on stage. That was true for a little while, but in the end, drinking made my writing suck, and drugs made me tell the same shitty story fifteen times and then burst into tears.

"I am grateful that I had those dubious crutches when I had them, and they simply aren't available to me anymore. For me, there is no way to deal with that but acceptance. I just accept that drugs and alcohol don't work for me, and that means I have to sit with my writing when it feels tough or slow or hard and just be all right with that. There is no alternative that I can think of.

"Usually I am really uncomfortable onstage and I just accept that that is part of my experience with the work that I do. As an alcoholic, I want everything to always be a joyride forever. I never want to feel discomfort, or awkwardness, or really have to work very hard, but those things are part of life's reality, and I can't drink a potion and make it not be so. I just accept it and trudge along, and really, my writing has gotten better from having to accept the challenge.

"I'm not really triggered to drink from being around alcohol, so being in bars doesn't bother me. I get triggered more by my emotions, not my environment. I really feel like that part of the Big Book that says we can go anywhere as long as we are working a good program has been really true for me. Usually I never want to drink, because my life has become so fucking amazing as a result of getting sober, I wouldn't want to jeopardize it. I never want it to go back to what it was."

I asked her what personal habits had changed for her since she got sober.

"I don't smoke as much. As it turns out, smoking is gross when I am actually sober and in my body. I do it if I'm really stressed, or sometimes on tour and performing a lot, because I feel compulsive. But I can feel how it gives me sinus infections so I have to be really careful. My coffee intake had to be shifted because I wasn't drinking it to pull myself out of a hangover. I started taking care of myself more once I got sober, and I still do. I work out a lot, and I care about my bedroom being nice. I also like having sex a lot more, and I am picky about my diet! Sometimes obsessively (with both sex and my diet). As an alcoholic I tend to do all things alcoholically (too much, trying to get high off it); sometimes it's a problem, and sometimes it's not. As long as I don't drink or do drugs, I let myself have as much of the rest of life as I want."

In response to my question about how addicts fit into the normal person's world:

"I don't think "normal" people are normal. Most people who aren't alcoholics qualify for a family support-type 12-Step program, in my opinion. I am taking the world's inventory here, but so what. I think that by working a spiritual program and taking responsibility for ourselves in the world we are setting an example for how to live a truly radical and awesome life. Even people who care about big political causes often treat the people around them, and their own selves, crappily. Working a program shows me how to live a life that really takes the best intentions of every political and spiritual discipline and puts it to work with little egomaniacal fanfare. I think most people could learn how to live better from anyone in any 12-Step program."

I asked her what inspiration she'd received outside of the official literature.

"A book called *Happy Hours: Alcohol in a Woman's Life* by Devon Jersild was helpful to me when I was trying to quit drinking but was too proud and scared to join a group. It helped ease me into the idea that I might be an actual alcoholic. I read a lot of Buddhist literature—basically everything Pema Chodron ever wrote is really helpful to me, as is the *Tao Te Ching*. I think Buddhism and 12-Step work have a lot of commonality, though I did try to just Buddha myself sober and found it did not work; in fact, then you're like one of those crazy alcoholic spiritual people, which is one of the most embarrassing types of nervous breakdowns; don't do it. There is a great book with the unfortunate title *Radical Acceptance: Embracing Your Life With the Heart of a Buddha* by Tara Brach that makes me cry every time I read it, so I can only read a bit at a time 'cause I hate crying. I like the *Living Sober* book too, 'cause it was written by a gay!

"If I honestly think about what will really happen if I drink (as opposed to what I want to happen if I drink), it stops me from picking up, because I know it only leads to me pooping my pants and crying in public, two of my least favorite things."

## MMORPGs

A lot of people approach me and say they are addicted to something. I know they're just trying to bond with me on some social level, but they come off as insulting. "You know what I'm addicted to? Shopping. I'm a shopaholic." or "I'm a chocoholic." This is ignorant in a way. You're not addicted to shopahol or chocohol. The sad part is, some people really are addicted to these things, to the point that they lose jobs, relationships, and their health because of it. But it's never people who are in a 12-Step program for debt or overeating that say those things to me. Then there are people who tell me they're addicted to their favorite TV program.

> 'You know what I'm addicted to? Shopping. I'm a shopaholic.' or 'I'm a chocoholic.' This is ignorant in a way. You're not addicted to shopahol or chocohol.

If you're addicted to a TV show, you would miss work to watch it and you would rewatch it hoping it ends differently. But one thing I heard of that I thought was in the joke-addicted category turned out not to be.

I've heard from parents and spouses that their loved ones were addicted to online gaming. I wasn't sure if they really meant the word addicted when they said it. Maybe it was one of those times when people used the word loosely. I've heard jokes made about Everquest and World of Warcraft, that people call them evercrack and warcrack. But what's the difference between the games being really good and them being addictive?

I'm not a hater on the games. I don't see much difference in coming home from work and watching TV until you crash out and playing video games for the same amount of time. Many Americans watch TV from the time they get home to the time they fall asleep. While it's not productive, I don't think it's necessarily debilitating. You can make the argument that the games are interactive. And online gaming is much more social than television.

The MMORPGs are a relatively new form of gaming. It started with RPGs, role-playing games. In an RPG, players assume roles and interact with other computer characters in the game to solve puzzles, complete quests, and improve their characters' abilities. RPGs generally took a long time to finish, but unlike many other video games, there was an end, an overall goal to reach. With the advent of online gaming, new areas and quests could be added throughout the life of the game. With the addition of other players, you can interact with other people rather than computer-controlled bots. The MMO stands for "massively multiplayer online," so MMORPG stands for "massively multiplayer online role playing game."

MMORPGs are a serious international business. The amount of revenue they bring in makes the industry a competitor with all other forms of entertainment, including movies, television, and sports. Players pay a monthly fee to play the game, and the number of players worldwide is in the millions.

I'm no newcomer to video games, but I hadn't had any first-hand experience with MMORPGs. I worked for a big console maker of video games for two years. I wrote the strategy guides that the 900 operators used to answer questions for callers. I went to work and played the same game for eight hours every day for five or six weeks, while taking notes on every minute aspect of the game. Then I got together with the others who were playing, and we put together the book on the game. A lot of my coworkers were into the early MMORPGs. That's when I first heard about them in detail.

The most hardcore gamers I knew were making fun of other people they knew. There were people who were losing relationships over the games they played. Not only were their significant others complaining about the time spent playing the game, the players were meeting other people and having cyber affairs. People were losing jobs over missed work time. People were undergoing physical changes with declining health and weight gain. There were tales of guys who peed in bottles so they didn't have to move away from the keyboard. At the time, I was more concerned with getting to the liquor store after work and drinking alone than going online and playing video games.

Newly sober, I had the problem of too much time on my hands. There are a lot of solutions to this problem. I eventually solved mine by getting back into writing, performing live, watching movies, and reading books. But for a few months, I checked out a very popular MMORPG.

In the first minutes of play, I gained my first level. In about ten more minutes, I had my next level. Twenty more minutes, the next. An hour, the next. I could see how it was going. I'd played enough RPGs to see this pattern. The first levels happen quickly. The later levels take exponentially longer to achieve. These diminishing returns are the same ones that happen physically with drugs and alcohol.

That first high is the classic drug euphoria. There are junkies and crackheads relentlessly chasing the first high. My later years of drinking weren't fun like my first years were, and I never knew why. Taking acid, mushrooms, or ecstasy at first requires a lot less to get high; I initially took only one hit of acid at a time, but soon was taking four or more, and while I did trip harder or longer, it was that first experience that was always the best.

In a lot of ways, the level gains in video games are the high, the reward for play. New abilities, new stats, and access to better gear all are the rewards that come after increasing amounts of gameplay. It takes longer and longer to achieve these rewards as play goes on. Even if you start a new character, getting to second level doesn't have the same reward as it did before. It's a kind of tolerance the gamer builds.

After a few months, the quests and the level gains became so long, I couldn't complete them in a casual gaming session. The options were to play for longer amounts of time for the same emotional result, or to play more often. Playing half a quest and coming back another day didn't work well for me because I quickly forgot my way around the game's landscape.

The game was really cool. There were many types of characters to play and a lot of further customization beyond that. It looked great, all the weapons, armor, and monsters. I played with people of all ages all over the world. Beyond the action of the killing, there was an in-game auction house where it was fun to buy and sell items. But in the end, I couldn't justify the time it would take to get what I wanted out of the game.

The time involved would have drastically changed my personal life. All of my solitary entertainment would have to be curtailed or eliminated from my life. Books, television, and movies would all go by the wayside. Would it creep into the time that I spent writing? Would I schedule social activities around it? Would I eliminate social activities because of it? I didn't take it that far. I canceled my account.

My main concern with the game in relation to the addict is transference. My personal opinion is that it has a low risk for addiction. But for the addict, we have to watch all the low risk categories closely. Something that's not very addictive for a regular person can really take hold of us quickly. I can really picture myself bottoming out on such a game. I think if these games had been around when I was a teenager, I may have turned to them for the unhealthy escape from life that led me to alcohol. But being born when I was, there wasn't much chance of my getting addicted to Duck Hunt or Excitebike. I found alcohol first, and even in the face of drugs, my first allegiance was to getting a drink in my hand. There was some kind of emotional loyalty that I had to it.

My second concern with the gaming is for the next generation of addicts, specifically the children of addicts. Our children are prone to be addicts themselves. While we're vigilant to the obvious dangers they face in drugs and alcohol, this one could sneak by most of us. Not only are our children prone to be addicts, this is a "drug" that is different from what their parents did. It's a way for them to rebel that we don't understand. Our

> **Our generation's version of dropping acid in a basement and watching a VHS tape of *The Wall* is their going online for a guild raid.**

generation's version of dropping acid in a basement and watching a VHS tape of *The Wall* is their going online for a guild raid.

My opinion doesn't have the authority of a listing in the DSM IV. MMORPGs are not officially addictive. But if even a small portion of a percentage of people are addicted to the games, with millions of people playing worldwide, there are a multitude of people suffering.

Hardcore gamers can experience:

- Building of a tolerance

- Difficulty cutting down playing time

- Social activities reorganizing around gameplay

- Extreme mood changes when forced with an inability to play

- Severe loss of sleep, trading the time for gameplay

These are all symptoms consistent with addiction.

If you or someone you know is lying about playing time, gaining significant amounts of weight because of playing, loses a job because of playing, or puts a relationship in jeopardy over playing, take it seriously. It's more than a game when it changes how you live your life.

# CHAPTER 10

# HOW ADDICTS CAN BE OF SERVICE TO NORMIES

**In the rooms, we** often talk about being of service. It's important to take commitments and be available to help others. Because 12-Step meetings are completely run by the members, if we didn't all know how to do every job, the meetings would fall apart eventually. We all must take turns in the various roles necessary to keep the meetings going. We also form support networks, not only in the form of sponsors and sponsees, but in the form of phone lists and homegroups. But service also extends outside of the meetings.

We can be of service to the rest of the world as well. Putting away chairs, showing up early to make coffee, and sweeping up cigarette butts off the sidewalk is our entry into service. Once you learn how to be of service to the group, try taking it to the outside world.

## Time to Give

When I was making amends, most of the people didn't want me to make up anything to them. Not being resentful grudge holders like myself, they weren't angry with me, and they held no long-term gripe. They had forgiven me. Instead of anger or hate, they had compassion for me. They told me how much it hurt them to see me ruining my life. They told me how worried I had made them. They told me it tore them up to see me so consistently depressed. It really reinforced how different their way of thinking was than mine and gave me emotional goals to work toward. Most of them told me that it was enough that I would turn my life around.

> **Once you learn how to be of service to the group, try taking it to the outside world.**

These amends were for instances that were minor for the most part. It was me becoming an angry drunk at a party or leaving a pissed off phone message on their machine. It usually involved some unfortunate social situation. I hadn't broken things or stolen from them. It was mostly hurt feelings. Some of them didn't remember the time I had caused a scene, even though I carried the shame for years.

For these people, I was determined to work a solid program. I was excited when I could run into them in public and tell them I had another month clean and sober or that I had completed another step. I wanted them to know I was serious and giving a real effort. That's where I thought the amends was.

I helped one of these friends empty out a storage space. It wasn't much of a move. It only took a couple of hours. But when we were done, he asked me if I was still going to meetings. I told him I was. He told me that this kind of help I was giving him was the kind of help he wouldn't have asked of me before. I hadn't been reliable or sober enough to help him move.

In my early thirties, most of my normal friends were married. Some were homeowners. Some had children. Almost all of them had full, busy, lives. I was living in a four-hundred-dollar-a-month room, which in San Francisco was barely big enough for my full-sized futon. I was working, but I had little else to do with my days. I was going to meetings and trying to get back into the performance scene. I hadn't thought why my friend had asked me to help. None of his other friends had the time to help him out.

The newly clean and sober have a lot of time on our hands. It's maddening to us. I've written elsewhere in this book about how to fill this time. But normal people can't find the time to do what they need to do in a day. They have stuff to do every day. Think about it. They have day planners and calendars, and they still can't get to it all.

That's where we can be of help. Especially if you're new in a program and you're looking to fill your days. Lend a hand to one of these people. Offer help. They likely won't ask because they take responsibility for their own lives. But if you offer, they may take you up on it.

### Moving

This is a big one. When you want to move, no one is around. Movers are expensive, and a lot of people are tapped out financially making the move to a new place. Offer to help during a move. Bring a program friend.

## Babysitting

Depending on your history, your friends may not want you around a child. You may act like one yourself. They may not be any less afraid that the house will catch on fire if you're in it. So be prepared for them to say no if you're sketchy. And they're the ones who determine if you're sketchy, not you. But if you're somewhat sane, watching someone's kid for a few hours makes certain errands runnable.

> **Addicts are good in a crisis. We don't fold. We've seen worse. We've fully exercised our survival skills.**

If your friends are new stay-at-home parents, they may be going a little crazy for lack of adult contact. I've spent time with some of my new father friends playing video games or watching football, and they were thrilled.

## Crisis Times

Addicts are good in a crisis. We don't fold. We've seen worse. We've fully exercised our survival skills. Normal people don't have nearly as much practice as we do in dealing with life's horrible surprises. We have an emotional threshold beyond all but a minor part of the population.

I have a graveyard full of dead friends. They've died of AIDS, overdoses, crime, and chaos. I know people who drank less than I did, used less than I did, who died from what they did. It's never easy, but it's not as hard on me as it is on others.

When one of my normal friends goes through a death in the family or among his friends, I make sure to be there. Especially with men because we don't have the emotional skill set to talk about this kind of thing with others. That first tragic death is so hard to handle. You can be there to listen, or just to sit with your friend. Some people want to talk, and some people want to take their mind off it. Just be there.

### Talking to Your Friends' Kids about Drugs

Hey there, Uncle Drunkypants! Time to have a little talk with your friend's kid who just got caught with a bag of weed. You'd be surprised how uncomfortable this makes normal people. They react badly to finding out their kid got high. It almost sounds cute to us hearing a teenager relating stories of getting loaded.

> **Hey there, Uncle Drunkypants! Time to have a little talk with your friend's kid who just got caught with a bag of weed.**

You'll also be able to tell the difference between a kid who took a hit off a joint and a kid who's swiping Oxycontin. Your friend's kid, if he knows you, will likely feel more comfortable telling you about hard stuff he is going through than talking to the parental units about it.

I throw this in with my Twelfth Step. It's service and being of help to others who are having trouble because of drugs and alcohol. It may not be at addiction levels, but it's still an area in which you are a self-taught expert.

# WHO HELPS THE SELF-HELPER?

**It's been weird breaking** into the world of self-help. Normally, I was around comedians, poets, and other performing artists. Then *Get Up* put me into a foreign world of self-help full of its own prejudices and discriminations.

The main misconception about self-help writers is that we're well-adjusted people with all the answers. I'm definitely not. I have a lot of answers, but I also have a lot more unanswered questions. I'm still a mess. I'm still working out a lot of issues. I have a sponsor; I do step work.

I'm not "fixed." I didn't solve all my problems. What I did do is build emotional and spiritual skill sets that help me deal with problems as they arise.

I'm not a self-help book kind of guy, except now I've written two of them. What I mean is, I don't read them. That's precisely why my editor approached me for the first book. They wanted me to write a self-help book for people who don't read self-help books.

Oh, there are a lot of people who read nothing but self-help books. I have met many of them now. They bought *Get Up* at my readings, telling me it's for their nephew who's a rock musician. They asked me if I'd read this book or what I thought of that author, and I had to tell them I had no idea what they were talking about.

I have a sponsor. He's a god-guy, and I'm a higher-power embracing atheist. He's very patient with me, and I am extremely grateful for him. He's done more good for me in the last year than any one person in my sobriety.

I do step work. New sponsor, new travels through the steps. I'm finding things I didn't find before, and finding other things inside me that I thought I had abandoned and let go of.

I still struggle with problems that I've been working on for years. I am not well. I am sick. If I waited till I had it all figured out, I wouldn't write the book. I'll be working on my problems until I die. The good news is that I've found a way to enjoy my life as long as it lasts.

# GLOSSARY

**When I first got** into the rooms, I heard a lot of little phrases and sayings. Some of them I could figure out, but others baffled me. It's like a secret coded language. People would blurt out some phrase or acronym and the room would crack up.

In time, some of them made more sense. The steps are commonly used as verbs: "I had to Ninth Step my dad." There are other things that are funny because they are common thoughts that lead to a conclusion the group can see coming, like: "I went back to drinking right as I got out of rehab, because this time I knew I wouldn't take it too far." Often I had to ask someone next to me what these things meant.

In case you're too shy to ask someone else, I'll spoil your fun here. I hope these explanations help keep you from being frustrated and accept the program stuff in spite of their weirdness.

**1-2-3 out:** Many people who get involved in a 12-Step program don't make it past the first three steps. There's a wall at the Fourth

Step that people don't seem to get over. The first three steps are acknowledgment and resignation to the program. It's easy to say but not as easy to live it. At the Fourth Step, action is required, if only at a personal level. It's impossible to complete the Fourth Step if the first three weren't done well. To do the Fourth, you must have resigned your will to a higher power as it says in Step Three. If you're resisting the Fourth Step, you still have too much of the addict's will living in your mind.

**90 in 90:** This is the idea that you will go to 90 meetings in the first 90 days of your sobriety/recovery. It's a really good idea. What happens is that you're forced to go to a bunch of different meetings to fill up the 90. There are as many kinds of meetings as there are kinds of bars. Just because you hated most of the bars in your town didn't mean you quit going to bars; you found other bars to go to. Once you hit that many meetings, you're going to find the ones you click with. You'll find someone you want to be your sponsor, and someone will ask you to be of service.

> **Aiming at the ground is how alkies drink. We are drinking to hit the floor.**

**Aiming at the ground:** Aiming at the ground is how alkies drink. We are drinking to hit the floor. We're not drinking to catch a buzz or enjoy a drink after dinner for digestion. We're drinking to get fucked up and fast. We're not done until our body gives out and we're lying on the ground.

This is the problem with us ever trying to "drink like normal people." We're not normal. We're way past normal. Normal people don't like that feeling of lying on the ground, unable to move.

**Alligator arms:** Someone with alligator arms can't reach his wallet, since his arms are apparently too short. This happens when big groups go out to eat together. There's always one guy who never seems to be able to pay. I've paid for a lot of newcomers, a lot of guys who live in a facility somewhere, and a lot of unemployed guys. I'll gladly pay for a lot more. But at some point, people need to take care of themselves. If they can't, feel free to lob this moniker on them.

**Bleeding deacons:** These are referenced in the official literature of 12-Step groups, in what's referred to as "The Twelve and Twelve." The term is generally used to describe negative speaking old-timers, those who speak up and say that new things won't work or that things aren't being done according to tradition. It's actually a corruption of an older term, *bleating deacon.* This term came from American Protestant Christianity and refers to a deacon who bleats negativity like a sheep. If you've ever heard a sheep bleat, you'll know exactly what this is about.

**Burning desire:** You'll hear them ask if there's a burning desire at the end of a meeting. This means that if you think you're going to drink or use after the meeting, then you should say something. By all means, use this opportunity, if you so feel. People will stop what they are doing and help you. However, it's for short shares and emergencies. Respect it, please.

**Detox, rehab, and the SLE:** I didn't know the difference between detox and rehab, and I had no idea what an SLE was. I heard it as "essilee." I didn't know it was an acronym. People in the rooms seem really familiar with them, and often know each other from being in one or more of these places.

*Detox* is where you go when you are kicking, when your body is still aching and going through withdrawals. It's used as a noun when it's the place you go, and as a verb when it's what you're going through. When you're detoxing in a detox facility, there are medical professionals there to monitor you in case something goes wrong. Alcohol detox can be fatal and should be monitored in such a place.

*Rehab* is where you get sent after you detox. Once you're out of immediate physical harm and freakouts, the detox facility is more than you need. But without going to rehab, most addicts and drunks go out and use again because they know nothing else to do.

When most people talk about rehab, they're talking about an inpatient facility. That's where the patients live onsite. There are many rules and few privileges, which must be earned and are easily taken away. The patients are forced to learn and maintain basic life skills. Rehabs range from exclusive retreats that are luxurious to drab masonry block-walled dormitories. If you can keep from getting drugs smuggled in and show off your minimal human qualities, you get to leave; your next move is sometimes the SLE.

An *SLE* is a "sober living environment." The SLE helps people learn more life skills and transition back into the real world.

Residents at an SLE can leave to go to work, but they still have curfews and rules to go by. They're still drug tested, but not as regularly as in rehab.

**Drink like normal people. Drink like a gentleman:** When normal people drink, they don't lose their jobs or wake up in other states. They don't get married to strangers. A gentleman doesn't get wasted at the company party and lash out at all his coworkers. Normal people can buy a six pack and only drink one beer. A gentleman can have a glass of wine and it doesn't lead to drinking the entire box.

I don't know of an alcoholic who didn't try this one out. It's a universal problem amongst us. We look around and see other people enjoying champagne at a wedding. They have one drink on the plane. They get wasted once a year on New Year's Eve.

> **When normal people drink, they don't lose jobs or wake up in other states. They don't get married to strangers.**

For that matter, normal people smoke pot whenever it's offered to them. They never seem to buy it, but they always smoke it when it's around. They don't have to go through bizarre rituals to pass drug tests. They never spend the whole day taking bong hits and watching the Cartoon Network.

We see other people just using or drinking a little, and it doesn't seem to ruin their lives. If we don't acknowledge that we're addicts and they're not, it's easy to rationalize a relapse. There are a lot of us who think we're "better." We're back to normal. We can drink like normal people or smoke pot like normal people, but this never works out.

**Dry drunk:** A dry drunk is someone who is not drinking anymore but has all the assholiness of someone who is. What's sometimes worse is that dry drunks are fully capable of acting on negative emotions and character defects, while the practicing drunk may soon forget his plans or be too wasted to carry them out.

While working security at bars, I've been swung at quite a bit, but only hit a few times. I've been hit more when one drunk tried to hit another. The best laid plans of mice and drunks often get fucked up along the way.

It's very common for people to wish the guy who quit drinking would start again. "I liked him better when he was drunk." That kind of thing.

Some people are more pleasant when they're stoned. Some people are more fun when they're drunk. Almost everyone is nicer on ecstasy. And no one at all is anything but annoying on cocaine. But these are only because they don't have the social mechanisms to be those ways without it. Anyone who you'd rather be around when he or she is drunk probably should quit.

**Fake it 'til you make it:** This should be on the cover of the official literature. Quitting is completely opposed by every cell in your body. Very little about 12-Step groups felt normal or even helpful at first. I kept going anyway. I didn't know what else to do. This, in essence, is fakin' it. It's okay that it seems weird, or that it seems as if it won't work, or even that you don't like it. Keep going. Keep trying. It's going to take some time before it feels right.

**Geographic, or pulling a geographic:** This is a term I've never heard from anyone who wasn't a program type. When I overhear it in a conversation, I know I'm eavesdropping on program talk.

When you pull a geographic, you are running from your problems. A good way to put it is going for a fresh start. It's really easy to watch other people's problems follow them from place to place. I like to remind people of the Buckaroo Banzai quote, "No matter where you go, there you are."

I think this also applies to addicts and alkies in the way we leave jobs and relationships, even if we're not moving to another town.

> **As long as you have the same resentments, fears, and defects of character, you're going to repeat your mistakes.**

It's that whole idea that you can start over, and this time you'll do things differently. As long as you have the same resentments, fears, and defects of character, you're going to repeat your mistakes.

**God doesn't give you anything more than you can handle:** As an atheist, I have a problem with this statement. My higher power is not something that has knowledge of what I can handle, and thus, cannot choose for me what I can and can't handle. But again, the sentiment can make sense for me. I turn it into "If you can't handle it, it's not your problem to deal with." Just as there are some powers greater than yourself, there are going to be some problems that are more than you can handle. Death, for instance, is something you can't have control of; it's bigger than you, and more powerful. I wouldn't want to consider death my higher power, but it definitely is a higher problem.

**If you hang out in a barbershop long enough, you're going to get a haircut:** This saying drives me nuts. Mainly because you're going to get a haircut eventually whether you hang out in the barbershop or not. It's said in relation to who you're spending your time with or where you hang out. When I was newly sober, I still went to bars because that's where poetry readings and comedians were. There were people who told me that would be the cause of my relapse. They have a point, but I hate hearing a situation relegated to this aphorism.

Find out where your triggers are and avoid those things. For most, living in a clean and sober household will be enough. I can avoid all kinds of temptation in public, as long as my living situation is healthy and stable.

I'm not going to avoid going to a party because people will be drinking. However, I will leave early once they get wasted. Not because it will make me want to drink, but because it gets boring for me. There also have been times I smelled a nice Scotch or saw someone dumping an eightball of coke on a coffee table when I left right away because of the temptation.

**Insanity is doing the same thing over and over again and expecting different results:** Insanity is many different things. There's a book called the DSM IV that is full of explanations of what sanity is. It's the desk reference for psychiatrists that is the size of a suitcase and is full of descriptions of every official mental illness. This definition isn't in there. But what's important to know is that this is the insanity that's referred to in Step Two when it mentions "restore us to sanity." By this definition of insanity, yes, I was most definitely insane. I argued for a while that I wasn't insane, and this wasn't a valid definition of insanity. Oh, if only a higher power could restore me from my stubbornness.

**Keep coming back:** This is a catchall response to shares that are weird, awkward, painful, or overly negative. When you hear this, your pain and sickness is being recognized, and you're not being judged; you're being accepted as you are. People may not agree with you, but they can sympathize with you and remember how they were when they first came in. It's the "good luck" or "break a leg" of the recovery world.

**Keep it simple (stupid):** You know what the white stuff in bird shit is? Bird shit. I've never heard that in a meeting. I've only heard that from one guy ever, a junior high basketball coach. That's what he'd tell us when we'd overthink something. He used to call a timeout to tell us to score more points than the other team. "You know what it takes to win, boys? A higher score than the other team." Yes, Coach Obvious was a big fan of keeping it simple. He also kept it stupid.

The whole recovery process can be summed up simply as: go to meetings, work the steps. It's a whole lot better if you get a sponsor, get commitments, and take part in the fellowship. There's a lot of official literature you can read as well. Don't get so wrapped up in your head and your life dissection that you forget the simple parts that work so well.

**Let go and let God:** I really like the sentiment here, but I hate how it's put. What it means is, let your higher power deal with things that are not your issues. However, I also think you shouldn't let God do for you what you can do for yourself.

**Luxury problems:** Trying to choose between buying the Bentley or the Rolls Royce is a luxury problem. If that's the biggest problem in your life, your life is fantastic. Some real problems are how do I protect myself and how do I feed myself? Drugs and alcohol put us in danger, and deprive us of basic nutrition. Once we have a serious habit, we need that stuff on a regular basis. That's a problem. It's a big problem when we don't have any money or a job, and we need the drugs.

> Don't get so wrapped up in your head and your life dissection that you forget the simple parts that work so well.

Most of our early recovery/sobriety problems are easy to see. We need a place to live. We need a job. We need to go to a meeting. We can deal with those. Once we get to another level, we're not prepared to deal with our luxury problems. Which apartment do we choose? Which car do we buy? Luxury problems can make us lose sight of the big picture in life.

When we get caught up in our luxury problems, it takes away from the attention we should be paying to living a righteous life.

**My worst day sober is better than my best day drunk:** My best days drunk were really fucking awesome, and I've had some shitty days sober. I kept drinking even though it was fucking up my life, because I was trying to have one of those awesome days again. I appreciate the sentiment, but it's just not true for me or most people. I can't blindly put all of my drunk time in the bad category, nor can I put my sober time in the good category. Overall, the last years of my drinking were a slow miserable slide into depression. And my best days sober have been the best days of my life. My best days drunk don't come close to my best days sober. I killed a bunch of good days by getting drunk and fucking them up.

**One is too many and a hundred is not enough:** For me, one was never enough. The same with a hundred. Nothing was enough. The first time I heard this, I objected. One was never too many. But the idea is that one just leads to more, and is, in essence, many drinks, like one really huge glass.

**Parole and halfway houses:** One aspect of parole that most Americans don't understand is that you can't get paroled unless you have a place to go, a viable address. Sometimes employment is required. I can't imagine how horrible it must be to be eligible for parole but unable to meet the conditions. For people without families or such contacts, there are halfway houses.

*Halfway houses* are halfway between being locked up and free. You're not incarcerated, but you can't quite come and go as you please either. There are frequent UA tests. There are strict curfews and regulations. Often there is a requirement to attend a 12-Step meeting, which is why you will eventually run into people from a halfway house.

> The pink cloud is a euphoric state where it looks like everything bad in life is in the past, and the future is nothing but rainbows and unicorns.

The people in halfway houses aren't always sure that drugs and alcohol are their problem, even if the reason for their incarceration was directly related to drugs and alcohol. Usually they're going to meetings because of a requirement, not because they've hit bottom yet.

**Pink cloud:** The pink cloud is what happens to people in the program when, for the first time in years, or maybe ever, shit starts working out. Life can be good, it seems, despite all previous thoughts to the contrary. The pink cloud is a euphoric state where it looks like everything bad in life is in the past, and the future is nothing but rainbows and unicorns.

I can't speak from experience here. I never got the pink cloud. Not everyone does. My first six months kinda sucked. But then again, I was isolating, going to meetings, but otherwise white knuckling it.

**Praise the lord and pass the ammunition:** This is one of my favorites. You might hear it as praise the lord and pass the recovery. Or praise the lord and pass the big book.

The saying goes back a long way. Some say it originated at the Alamo. The idea is that praying is a good idea, but you also have to take action. You can't just sit around and wait for your higher power to do everything.

**Stinkin' thinkin':** This is in reference to your entire mental process. You can't come to good conclusions because your entire reasoning system is flawed. You think like a drunk, even sober, and therefore, you will act like one. This is much like a dry drunk. You'll be accused of stinkin' thinkin' when you give someone a reason for what you've done or what you're about to do.

**Take the cotton out of your ears and stick it in your mouth:** Shut up and listen. This is another aphorism that people think is clever but is really insulting. What, my opinion matters nothing? But eventually, you will meet someone who talks such a line of shit that you will find these words coming up your throat. I prefer reminding such people about the *Karate Kid* line, "Teacher say, student do. No questions."

**You can complain in one hand and shit in the other:** The last part of that statement is . . . "and see which one fills up first." That's the whole saying, but it's often truncated. If I hadn't heard the whole saying first, I would've had no idea what this means. Action is better than talking. Complaining gets you nothing. Shitting in your hand gets you a handful of shit. Which should be its own aphorism. At least the action will get you a result.

**Wet brain:** There's an actual clinical diagnosis for this. The medical name is Wernicke-Korsakoff Syndrome. It's permanent brain damage brought on by a thiamine (vitamin B1) deficiency, which occurs from poor diet or from damaging the internal organs that process thiamine from food. It's a very serious and sometimes fatal syndrome.

This term is bandied about in the rooms as an excuse for any lapse in brain function. "I'm too wet-brained to remember that." Some people think they have it or say other people have it. But clinically, it's much more intense than just forgetting to show up early to set up chairs before the meeting.

It's used also for people who still look a little drunk when they're sober. This is similar to permaburn for stoners and permatweak for meth users. Ninety-nine percent of the time when you hear the words "wet brain," you're hearing nothing more than a slang term.

**White knuckle:** White knuckling is the term for staying sober, but it's painful. Grip something really tight, and your knuckles go white. It's the lack of blood in the knuckles. It can also be used as "white knuckler," someone who stays sober this way.

Why is it painful? The white knuckler doesn't work steps or have a sponsor. Some white knucklers have been known to go to meetings, but they don't participate, fellowship, or do any service work.

White knuckling often works. However, you'll be miserable. All the character defects you have that make you want to drink will still be there. You'll constantly be thinking of drinking, and constantly not be drinking. You will spend all day not drinking. White knuckling can get you through a harsh time or a bad moment, but you'll feel like crap the whole time.

I've had long periods of white knuckling. I was sad, angry, confused, jaded, bitter, and jealous. But I didn't drink, which is the most important thing. The second most important thing is that I started up a good program again.

# ALSO BY BUCKY SINISTER

*Get Up: A 12-Step Guide to Recovery for Misfits, Freaks & Weirdos*

*King of the Roadkills*
*Whiskey and Robots*
*All Blacked Out & Nowhere to Go*

Comedy CD:
*What Happens in Narnia, Stays in Narnia*

Chapbooks:
*12 Bowls of Glass*
*Asphalt rivers*
*A Friend and a Killer*
*Symphony of the Damned*
*NASCAR*
*Blackout Poems for Drunk Readers*
*Tragedy and Bourbon*
*Fever Dreams*
*Angels We Have Heard While High*

Poetry Record:
*Sensitive Badass*

# ABOUT THE AUTHOR

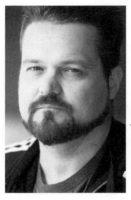

Photo by Ameen Belbahri

**Bucky Sinister** is a recovering alcoholic and addict. He is the author of several books of poetry and *Get Up: A 12-Step Guide to Recovery for Misfits, Freaks & Wierdos*. He lives in San Francisco.

Visit him on the web at *www.buckysinister.com*.

# To Our Readers

Conari Press, an imprint of Red Wheel/Weiser, publishes books on topics ranging from spirituality, personal growth, and relationships to women's issues, parenting, and social issues. Our mission is to publish quality books that will make a difference in people's lives – how we feel about ourselves and how we relate to one another. We value integrity, compassion, and receptivity, both in the books we publish and in the way we do business.

Our readers are our most important resource, and we appreciate your input, suggestions, and ideas about what you would like to see published.

Visit our website *www.redwheelweiser.com* where you can subscribe to our newsletters and learn about our upcoming books, exclusive offers, and free downloads.

You can also contact us at info@redwheelweiser.com.

Conari Press
an imprint of Red Wheel/Weiser, LLC
500 Third Street, Suite 230
San Francisco, CA 94107